Ethnicity and Psychopharmacology

Review of Psychiatry Series
John M. Oldham, M.D., and
Michelle B. Riba, M.D.
Series Editors

Ethnicity and Psychopharmacology

EDITED BY

Pedro Ruiz, M.D.

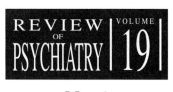

REVIEW OF PSYCHIATRY | VOLUME 19

No. 4

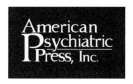

American Psychiatric Press, Inc.

Washington, DC
London, England

Note: The authors have worked to ensure that all information in this book concerning drug dosages, schedules, and routes of administration is accurate as of the time of publication and consistent with standards set by the U.S. Food and Drug Administration and the general medical community. As medical research and practice advance, however, therapeutic standards may change. For this reason and because human and mechanical errors sometimes occur, we recommend that readers follow the advice of a physician who is directly involved in their care or the care of a member of their family.

Books published by the American Psychiatric Press, Inc., represent the views and opinions of the individual authors and do not necessarily represent the policies and opinions of the Press or the American Psychiatric Association.

Copyright © 2000 American Psychiatric Press, Inc.
03   02   01   00   4   3   2   1

ALL RIGHTS RESERVED
Manufactured in the United States of America on acid-free paper

American Psychiatric Press, Inc.
1400 K Street, NW
Washington, DC 20005
www.appi.org

The correct citation for this book is

Ruiz P (ed.): *Ethnicity and Psychopharmacology* (Review of Psychiatry Series, Vol. 19, No. 4; Oldham JO and Riba MB, series eds.). Washington, DC, American Psychiatric Press, 2000

Library of Congress Cataloging-in-Publication Data
A CIP record is available from the Library of Congress (LC Control Number: 00024854).

British Library Cataloguing in Publication Data
A CIP record is available from the British Library.

Review of Psychiatry Series ISSN 1041-5882

Contents

Contributors

Gregory E. Gray, M.D., Ph.D.
Professor and Chairman, Department of Psychiatry and Human Behavior, Charles R. Drew University of Medicine and Science; Director, Augustus F. Hawkins Community Mental Health Center, Martin Luther King Jr./Drew Medical Center, Los Angeles, California

William B. Lawson, M.D., Ph.D., F.A.P.A.
Professor of Psychiatry, Indiana University School of Medicine; Chief, Psychiatry Service, Roudebush Veterans Administration Medical Center, Indianapolis, Indiana

Keh-Ming Lin, M.D., M.P.H.
Professor of Psychiatry, UCLA School of Medicine, Department of Psychiatry, Harbor-UCLA Medical Center, Torrance, California

Ricardo Mendoza, M.D.
Clinical Professor of Psychiatry, UCLA School of Medicine, Department of Psychiatry, Harbor-UCLA Medical Center, Torrance, California

John M. Oldham, M.D.
Director, New York State Psychiatric Institute; Dollard Professor and Acting Chairman, Department of Psychiatry, Columbia University College of Physicians and Surgeons, New York, New York

Edmond H. Pi, M.D.
Professor and Executive Vice Chairman, Department of Psychiatry and Human Behavior, Charles R. Drew University of Medicine and Science; Associate Director, Augustus F. Hawkins Community Mental Health Center, Martin Luther King Jr./Drew Medical Center, Los Angeles, California

Michelle B. Riba, M.D.
Clinical Associate Professor of Psychiatry and Associate Chair for Education and Academic Affairs, Department of Psychiatry, University of Michigan Health System, Ann Arbor, Michigan

Pedro Ruiz, M.D.
Professor and Vice Chair, Department of Psychiatry and Behavioral Sciences, University of Texas Medical School at Houston, Houston, Texas

David R. Small, M.B.A.

Executive Administrator, Harris County Psychiatric Center, Department of Psychiatry and Behavioral Sciences, University of Texas Medical School at Houston, Houston, Texas

Michael W. Smith, M.D.

Associate Professor of Psychiatry, UCLA School of Medicine, Department of Psychiatry, Harbor-UCLA Medical Center, Torrance, California

Roy V. Varner, M.D.

Professor and Medical Director, Harris County Psychiatric Center, Department of Psychiatry and Behavioral Sciences, University of Texas Medical School at Houston, Houston, Texas

Introduction to the Review of Psychiatry Series

John M. Oldham, M.D.
Michelle B. Riba, M.D., Series Editors

2000 REVIEW OF PSYCHIATRY SERIES TITLES

- *Learning Disabilities: Implications for Psychiatric Treatment*
  EDITED BY LAURENCE L. GREENHILL, M.D.
- *Psychotherapy for Personality Disorders*
  EDITED BY JOHN G. GUNDERSON, M.D., AND GLEN O. GABBARD, M.D.
- *Ethnicity and Psychopharmacology*
  EDITED BY PEDRO RUIZ, M.D.
- *Complementary and Alternative Medicine and Psychiatry*
  EDITED BY PHILIP R. MUSKIN, M.D.
- *Pain: What Psychiatrists Need to Know*
  EDITED BY MARY JANE MASSIE, M.D.

The advances in knowledge in the field of psychiatry and the neurosciences in the last century can easily be described as breathtaking. As we embark on a new century and a new millennium, we felt that it would be appropriate for the 2000 Review of Psychiatry Series monographs to take stock of the state of that knowledge at the interface between normality and pathology. Although there may be nothing new under the sun, we are learning more about not-so-new things, such as how we grow and develop; who we are; how to differentiate between just being different from one another and being ill; how to recognize, treat, and perhaps prevent illness; how to identify our unique vulnerabilities; and how to deal with the inevitable stress and pain that await each of us.

In the early years of life, for example, how can we tell whether a particular child is just rowdier, less intelligent, or more adventuresome than another child—or is, instead, a child with a learning or behavior disorder? Clearly, the distinction is crucial, because newer and better treatments that now exist for early-onset disorders can smooth the path and enhance the chances for a solid future for children with such disorders. Yet, inappropriately labeling and treating a rambunctious but normal child can create problems rather than solve them. Greenhill and colleagues guide us through these waters, illustrating that a highly sophisticated methodology has been developed to make this distinction with accuracy, and that effective treatments and interventions are now at hand.

Once we have successfully navigated our way into early adulthood, we are supposed to have a pretty good idea (so the advice books say) of who we are. Of course, this stage of development does not come easy, nor at the same time, for all. Again, a challenge presents itself—that is, to differentiate between widely disparate varieties of temperament and character and when extremes of personality traits and styles should be recognized as disorders. And even when traits are so extreme that little dispute exists that a disorder is present, does that disorder represent who the person is, or is it something the individual either inherited or developed and might be able to overcome? In the fifth century B.C., Hippocrates described different personality types that he proposed were correlated with specific "body humors"; this ancient principle remains quite relevant, though the body humors of today are neurotransmitters. How low CNS serotonin levels need to be, for example, to produce disordered impulsivity is still being determined, yet new symptom-targeted treatment of such conditions with SSRIs is now well accepted. What has been at risk as the neurobiology of personality disorders has become increasingly understood is the continued recognition of the importance of psychosocial treatments for these disorders. Gunderson and Gabbard and their colleagues review the surprisingly robust evidence for the effectiveness of these approaches, including new uses and types of cognitive-behavioral and psychoeducational methods.

It is not just differences in personality that distinguish us from one another. Particularly in our new world of global communication and population migration, ethnic and cultural differences are more often part of life in our own neighborhoods than just exotic and unfamiliar aspects of faraway lands. Despite great strides overcoming fears and prejudices, much work remains to be done. At the same time, we must learn more about ways that we are different (not better or worse) genetically and biologically, because uninformed ignorance of these differences leads to unacceptable risks. Ruiz and colleagues carefully present what we now know and do not know about ethnicity and its effects on pharmacokinetics and pharmacodynamics.

An explosion of interest in and information about wellness—not just illness—surrounds us. How to achieve and sustain a healthy lifestyle, how to enhance successful aging, and how to benefit from "natural" remedies saturate the media. Ironically, although this seems to be a new phenomenon, the principles of complementary or alternative medicine are ancient. Some of our oldest and most widely used medications are derived from plants and herbs, and Eastern medicine has for centuries relied on concepts of harmony, relaxation, and meditation. Again, as the world shrinks, we are obligated to be open to ideas that may be new to us but not to others and to carefully evaluate their utility. Muskin and colleagues present a careful analysis of the most familiar and important components of complementary and alternative medicine, presenting a substantial database of information, along with tutorials on non-Western (hence nontraditional to us) concepts and beliefs.

Like it or not, life presents us with stress and pain. Pain management has not typically figured into mainstream psychiatric training or practice (with the exception of consultation-liaison psychiatry), yet it figures prominently in the lives of us all. Massie and colleagues provide us with a primer on what psychiatrists should know about the subject, and there is a great deal indeed that we should know.

Many other interfaces exist between psychiatry as a field of medicine, defining and treating psychiatric illnesses, and the rest of medicine—and between psychiatry and the many paths of the life cycle. These considerations are, we believe, among our top priorities as we begin the new millennium, and these volumes provide an in-depth review of some of the most important ones.

Foreword

Pedro Ruiz, M.D.

The field of ethnopsychopharmacology has gained much respect and recognition during the last two to three decades. Several factors are responsible for this situation, including the maturity and growth of cultural psychiatry (Ruiz 1998), the recent expansion of ethnic minority populations in the United States (Ruiz 1995), the scientific advancement and acceptance of the field of ethnopsychopharmacology as a result of research efforts (Lin et al. 1995), and the recognition of the importance of ethnicity, culture, and race in the *Diagnostic and Statistical Manual of Mental Disorders,* 4th Edition (DSM-IV) (American Psychiatric Association 1994).

Traditionally, five human races have been recognized (Karlow 1992). Members of three of them (the Caucasoid, Mongoloid, and Negroid races) represent the largest groups in the world's population, and San (Bushmen) and Australian aborigines make up smaller population groups. However, each of these five large races is composed of subgroups, and many of these subgroups are racially mixed. Therefore, it is more practical and useful to divide the population on the basis of genetic differences.

At the core of ethnopsychopharmacology are three basic mechanisms: pharmacokinetics, pharmacodynamics, and pharmacogenetics. Pharmacokinetics deals with the fate and distribution of drugs in biological organisms, including humans. Pharmacokinetic processes are based on absorption, distribution, metabolism (biotransformation), and excretion of drugs. These four basic processes are the ones that determine the concentration of psychopharmacological agents in the blood. Metabolism, in particular, plays a very important role in this regard. Pharmacokinetic mechanisms have been extensively investigated with respect to cross-ethnic and interindividual variations in drug responses (Karlow 1992).

Pharmacodynamics addresses the way in which psychopharmacological agents affect the biological organism, that is, by interacting with receptors that bind with both endogenous and exogenous substances. Extensive cross-ethnic and individual variability exists in this regard (Karlow 1992). Pharmacogenetics deals with genetic and environmental factors that control and/or influence drug-metabolizing enzymes (Karlow 1992).

Besides these three basic mechanisms, which are central to the field of ethnopsychopharmacology, there are also nonbiological elements that can influence the way in which individuals respond to medications. These elements are compliance factors, placebo effects, stress, social support, personality styles, and physician prescribing patterns (Karlow 1992).

Pharmacogenetically, differences in the genetic structure of the drug-metabolizing enzymes can explain, in large measure, the ethnic variations that have been reported in psychopharmacological responses (Smith and Mendoza 1996). The cytochrome P450 (CYP) enzyme system is the main pathway of drug metabolism in humans. These enzymes are responsible for the metabolism of most psychopharmacological agents. Ethnic differences in drug metabolism appear to be related to the polymorphic variation of the same enzyme, that is, to the different forms of the same enzyme. These polymorphic differences may be the result of the evolutionary forces that have an impact on the CYP system (Smith and Mendoza 1996).

The two most extensively investigated CYP enzymes are debrisoquin hydroxylase H (CYP2D6) and mephenytoin hydroxylase (CYP2C19). These two enzymes are responsible for the metabolism of many commonly used medications, such as cardiovascular, analgesic, and psychopharmacological agents (Smith and Mendoza 1996). Depending on his or her enzyme polymorphism, an individual can be categorized as an extensive metabolizer or a poor or slow metabolizer. In general, poor or slow metabolizers tend to have higher blood levels of psychopharmacological agents. In these cases, toxic levels of psychopharmacological agents and thus increased severity of side effects are commonly observed, even when standard doses are prescribed (Smith and Mendoza 1996). The psychopharmacological agents metabolized by the CYP2D6 enzyme are most of the antidepressant and neuroleptic agents (Llerena et al. 1996). The psychopharmacological agents metabolized by the CYP2C19 enzyme are the benzodiazepines and some of the tricyclic antidepressants (Lin et al. 1995).

Most psychotropic agents are highly lipophilic and rely on plasma proteins for transport through the blood (Reidenberg and Erill 1986). Variations in the plasma concentrations of these drug-binding transport proteins can influence the effect of psychopharmacological agents, by changing the free fraction of these drugs and therefore the unbound (free) psychopharmacological concentrations in the plasma (Levy and Moreland 1984; Routledge 1986). The free (unbound) fraction is the only part of the drug that is pharmacologically active and capable of crossing the blood-brain barrier; therefore, changes in the concentration of the drug-binding protein are of high clinical relevance. Moreover, ethnic variations have been reported not only in the structure of drug-binding plasma protein but in its quantity as well (Lin et al. 1995). Body size and composition also often vary across ethnic groups. Therefore, the volume of distribution of psychotropic drugs can also vary, particularly with drugs that are lipophilic. Additionally, toxins, pharmaceutical agents, sex hormones, tobacco, alcohol, caffeine, and dietary factors can have an effect on the P450 enzymes (Lin et al. 1995).

Culture also plays a major role. For instance, physician bias, placebo effects, compliance factors, and patient beliefs and expectations all can influence the clinical effects of psychotropic agents (Smith et al. 1993). It has been reported that because of psychiatric practitioner bias, severe psychiatric illnesses are often diagnosed in African American patients, who are then prescribed high doses of neuroleptics (Price et al. 1985). It has also been reported that Caucasians tend to be more responsive than non-Caucasians to placebo (Escobar and Tuason 1980).

In this book, we address the most relevant theoretical and clinical aspects of ethnopsychopharmacology. We also expect to advance the field of ethnopsychopharmacology well into the twenty-first century.

In the opening chapter, Drs. Keh-Ming Lin and Michael W. Smith present an extensive review of the issues surrounding the influence of cultural and ethnic forces on psychotropic responses.

The literature reviewed in this chapter clearly depicts the role of ethnic and cultural factors in the practice of psychopharmacology. Age and sex factors also need to be examined in this context. The ultimate goal, as set forth in this chapter, is an integrative approach in which both ethnic or cultural diversity and biological diversity are taken into account and treatment is tailored to specific individual characteristics.

In the second chapter, Dr. William B. Lawson describes how culture, social perception, biological factors, and access to care affect psychopharmacological treatment and responses among African American patients. Noteworthy in this respect is that current psychopharmacological practices lead to the prescription of higher doses of antipsychotic medications in black populations. There is a tendency to overdiagnose psychotic disorders and underdiagnose affective and anxiety disorders among African Americans. Likewise, black perceptions of the current mental health system in this country, as well as the attitudes of Caucasian psychiatric practitioners vis-à-vis African American patients, also have an impact on psychopharmacological prescribing practices. The chapter includes a discussion of the potential increase of side effects of psychopharmacological agents in African American populations due to pharmacokinetic, pharmacodynamic, and pharmacogenetic factors. Dr. Lawson outlines the benefits of newer psychopharmacological agents among black patients, benefits that are the result of better tolerance, fewer side effects, and increased efficacy. The chapter concludes with cautions about limitations in access to psychiatric care because of social policy and the cost of psychopharmacological agents.

In the third chapter, Drs. Ricardo Mendoza and Michael W. Smith focus on the psychopharmacological treatment of Hispanic patients in the United States and also underline the fact that, given the growth rate of the country's Hispanic population, American psychiatrists will be treating increasing numbers of Hispanic patients. Additionally, current data are available that support the notion of genetic variation among Hispanic subgroups. Drs. Mendoza and Smith also review the mechanisms involved in the biotransformation of psychoactive compounds—particularly the pharmacogenetics of the CYP drug-metabolizing–enzyme system—among Hispanics. There is an extensive review of reports of clinical experience related to the psychopharmacological treatment of Hispanics. Finally, some guidelines are offered geared toward minimizing cultural barriers in the psychiatric treatment of Hispanic populations and thus optimizing psychopharmacotherapeutic responses.

In the fourth chapter, Drs. Edmond H. Pi and Gregory E. Gray review the pharmacokinetics, pharmacodynamics, and sociocultural influences on the psychotropic responses among Asian American populations. Particular consideration is given to antipsychotics, antidepressants, benzodiazepines, and lithium. The authors stress the importance of prescribing the lowest possible effective dose, to minimize untoward side effects and thus ensure treatment compliance.

In the fifth and final chapter, Drs. Roy V. Varner and Pedro Ruiz and David R. Small, M.B.A., address the need for investigational studies focusing on pharmacokinetic, pharmacodynamic, and pharmacogenetic factors in the public psychiatric sector. After all, it is in the public sector that most of the ethnic or cultural minority groups in the United States receive their psychiatric care. Also reviewed are the results of several studies of responses to antidepressants and neuroleptics by multiethnic populations treated in the public sector.

In summary, our intention in these five chapters is to discuss the most recent advances in ethnopsychopharmacology, as well as to portray the future of the field. In recent years, sustained research efforts have led to great progress in ethnopsychopharmacology, but the field is very young and there are many more scientific advances to be made.

I thank all of the authors who joined me in accepting the challenge of producing this important contribution to ethnopsychopharmacology. I also thank Drs. John M. Oldham and Michelle B. Riba, editors of the Review of Psychiatry Series, for their vision in dedicating a book to such a significant area of psychiatry. We hope that this book on ethnicity and psychopharmacology will be useful to psychiatric practitioners, educators, and investigators.

References

American Psychiatric Association: Diagnostic and Statistical Manual of Mental Disorders, 4th Edition. Washington, DC, American Psychiatric Association, 1994

Escobar J, Tuason V: Antidepressant agents: a cross-cultural study. Psychopharmacol Bull 16:49–52, 1980

Kalow W (ed): Pharmacogenetics of Drug Metabolism. New York, Pergamon, 1992

Levy R, Moreland T: Rationale for monitoring free drug levels. Clin Pharmacokinet 1 (suppl):1-9, 1984

Lin K-M, Anderson D, Poland RE: Ethnicity and psychopharmacology: bridging the gap. Psychiatr Clin North Am 18:635–647, 1995

Llerena A, Cobaleda J, Martinez C, et al: Interethnic differences in drug metabolism: influence of genetic and environmental factors on debrisoquine hydroxylation phenotype. Eur J Drug Metab Pharmacokinet 21:129–138, 1996

Price N, Glazer W, Morgenstern H: Race and the use of fluphenazine decanoate. Am J Psychiatry 142:1491–1492, 1985

Reidenberg M, Erill S: Drug-Protein Binding. New York, Oxford University Press, 1986

Routledge P: The plasma protein binding of basic drugs. Br J Clin Pharmacol 22:499–506, 1986

Ruiz P: Assessing, diagnosing, and treating culturally diverse individuals: a Hispanic perspective. Psychiatr Q 66:329–341, 1995

Ruiz P: New clinical perspectives in cultural psychiatry. Journal of Practical Psychiatry and Behavioral Health 4:150–156, 1998

Smith MW, Mendoza RP: Ethnicity and pharmacogenetics. Mt Sinai J Med 63:285–290, 1996

Smith MW, Lin K-M, Mendoza R: Nonbiological issues affecting psychopharmacotherapy: cultural considerations, in Psychopharmacology and Psychobiology of Ethnicity. Edited by Lin K-M, Poland RE, Nakasaki G. Washington, DC, American Psychiatric Press, 1993, pp 37–58

Chapter 1

Psychopharmacotherapy in the Context of Culture and Ethnicity

Keh-Ming Lin, M.D., M.P.H.
Michael W. Smith, M.D.

The advent of the modern era of psychopharmacology in the early 1950s represented one of the most significant and dramatic milestones in the history of psychiatry and mental health. In the last half century, this relatively young field has not only provided a myriad of increasingly safe and efficacious intervention methods but also invigorated research in neuroscience and substantially enriched our understanding of the function of the brain, both in normal and abnormal conditions (Bloom et al. 1995). In addition, by enabling a large number of severely disturbed patients to move from confined settings to community living, psychopharmacological advances contributed toward the development of effective psychosocial rehabilitative programs and thereby played a pivotal role in the reshaping of the mental health care delivery system.

The power of these modern-day wonder drugs is persuasively demonstrated by the fact that within a few years of their discovery, they were introduced into practically all geographic areas of the world and quickly became the mainstay for the care of mentally ill persons in all societies (Lin et al. 1993). This is in sharp contrast with other psychiatric traditions that originated in Western countries (e.g., dynamic psychiatry), whose penetration into most non-Western societies has been slow and limited. The effectiveness and specificity of different classes of psychotropics often seem to tran-

Supported in part by National Institute of Mental Health Research Center on the Psychobiology of Ethnicity Grant no. MH47193.

scend cultural and ethnic boundaries (Lin and Cheung 1999; Lin et al. 1993). It appears that, in general, psychiatric medications are widely accepted and are regarded as useful and helpful by patients and their families, irrespective of their cultural backgrounds.

However, as an outgrowth of the psychiatric profession's accumulated experiences in the practice of psychopharmacotherapy in divergent cultural and ethnic settings, numerous reports of cross-cultural or cross-ethnic variations in psychotropic responses also have been appearing in the literature, reports collectively indicating that culture and ethnicity often significantly influence aspects of psychopharmacotherapeutic practices (Lin and Poland 1995). Until most recently, practically all psychiatric medications were developed and tested in North America and Western Europe (in studies predominantly involving young white males), where scientifically based information regarding the extent of such influences has been unsystematic and scattered (Lin et al. 1999). However, both theoretical considerations and data derived from divergent fields make it increasingly clear that these issues, like issues concerning age and sex, require much more careful attention, both in research and in clinical practice, than was previously thought necessary (Jensvold et al. 1996).

Pitfall of the Color-Blind Approach

Substantial individual variation in drug responses is the rule rather than the exception. Although the current understanding of such remarkable variability remains incomplete, much is determined by genetic and environmental factors that are often associated with or are significantly influenced by an individual's origin or lifestyle or other sociodemographic variables. Given that this is the case, it is remarkable that clinicians and researchers have tended to ignore the importance of such influences. Several major reasons might be responsible for this. There has been a profound tendency in psychiatry to equate biology with universality and to regard variations in responses to biomedical interventions as "noise." Also, a history of recurrent racist misinterpretation, distortion, and/or outright fabrication of scientific data has made

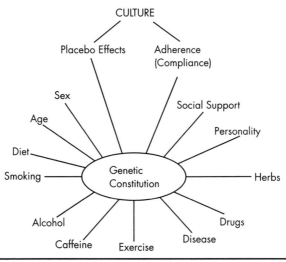

Figure 1–1. Factors affecting drug response.

any discussion of biological diversity among people suspect and anxiety-ridden. Finally, when taken out of the context of the often equally substantial individual variability that exists in any population groups, findings of ethnic differences run the risk of being interpreted simplistically and stereotypically. Because of these and other reasons, ethnic variations in pharmacological responses have often been regarded with suspicion and are not taken seriously (Lin et al. 1999).

However, as is clear from Figure 1–1, virtually all factors affecting pharmacological responses are significantly influenced by culture and ethnicity. As will be described in greater detail later, patterns of genetic polymorphism, often with substantial ethnic variation, exist in a large number of genes controlling the metabolism of drug-metabolizing enzymes as well as receptors and transporters believed to be targets of pharmaceutical agents. In addition, the expression of these genes is often significantly modified by a large number of environmental factors, including diet and exposure to various substances (e.g., tobacco). Of even greater importance, the success of any therapy, including pharmacotherapy, depends on the participation of the patient as well as the nature and quality of the interaction between the clinician and the patient. The importance of culture in this regard is paramount.

Cultural Context of Psychopharmacotherapy

Perhaps one of the biggest problems in contemporary medical healing practice is its tendency to focus—often exclusively—on technological, biomedical interventions (Kleinman 1988). This tendency frequently obscures the fact that treatment almost always takes place in the context of interactions among individuals. In these interactions, all participants bring into play their own knowledge, predispositions, values, priorities, modes of thinking, and belief systems. Further, perhaps reflecting the bias of Western culture, these interactions are traditionally discussed in terms of the relationship between the clinician and the patient (Marsella et al. 1985). However, in reality, neither the patient nor the clinician acts in isolation. No matter how isolated, patients almost always make decisions within the context of real or imagined input from people around them. Clinicians, too, as members of professional groups, are profoundly influenced by the opinions of their peers and prevailing ideologies in the field. As medical care in most societies becomes increasingly organized, institutional control over and influences on the practice of physicians and other health care professionals become progressively more prominent. In addition, the pharmaceutical industry has a powerful influence on clinicians' prescription behaviors as well as researchers' foci and priorities. Thus, although most pharmacotherapeutic decisions may appear technically based and straightforward, on closer look they are always found to be affected by sociocultural factors that both the patient and the clinician have brought into the transaction (Smith et al. 1993).

Despite their apparent significance, these contextual issues have rarely received adequate attention from clinicians and researchers. Often they are regarded as "noise" or even a nuisance. Consequently, there has been a dearth of information regarding the nature and determinants of related issues, such as adherence (compliance) and the "expectation effect" (including the placebo effect). Even less is known about how sociocultural factors affect these processes. Although much awaits further clarification, the extant literature in aggregate does support the suggestion that social and cultural forces play a major role in determining the expectations and behaviors of both clinicians and patients. These in turn affect the process and outcome of treatments.

Clinician Attitudes

A large body of literature indicates that patients' cultural or ethnic backgrounds significantly determine the way clinicians conceptualize and label their problems, which in turn dictates the choices for therapeutic intervention (Mezzich et al. 1995). Using case vignettes that were identical except for ethnic group identification, investigators in a number of studies demonstrated that significantly more severe diagnoses were made in cases identical in every other aspect if the patients were identified as belonging to ethnic minority groups (Gaw 1993; Lopez 1989). Paralleling such a tendency, African American psychiatric patients have been significantly more likely than their Caucasian counterparts to have their conditions diagnosed as schizophrenia (Littlewood 1992; Lopez 1989). Interestingly, in studies in which patients were reassessed with the use of structured interviews, such differences largely disappeared, further supporting the thesis that this differential diagnostic pattern is largely determined by variables related to clinician bias rather than to patients' clinical conditions (Adebimpe 1981; Marquez et al. 1985; Mukherjee et al. 1983; Roukema et al. 1984). It is likely that similar biases led to the pervasive use of higher doses of neuroleptics in treating African American patients, irrespective of diagnosis. Studies have also shown that African American patients were more likely than their Caucasian counterparts to be treated with depot neuroleptics, presumably because of a general perception that African Americans have problems with compliance (Price et al. 1985; Strickland et al. 1991).

The potential consequence of these diagnostic and treatment biases may be far from innocuous. Several large-scale studies have documented that the rate of tardive dyskinesia also is significantly higher in African Americans (Morgenstern and Glazer 1993; Sramek et al. 1991; Swartz et al. 1997). Although other reasons for this heightened risk of tardive dyskinesia among African Americans have not been ruled out, it is very likely that their increased exposure to neuroleptics accounts for at least part of this risk.

The effect of clinicians' attitudes on the treatment of other ethnic minority groups has been less well documented (Pi et al. 1993). However, given that difficulties in psychiatric assessment and management planning usually grow in proportion to cultural and social distance between clinicians and patients, it is reasonable to expect that misdiagnosis and inappropriate use of psychotropics also represent significant problems in clinical settings where patients are treated by clinicians who are not familiar with their cultural backgrounds.

Adherence

The magnitude of the problem of noncompliance with psychotropic treatment, commonly in the range of 20%–90%, has been well documented (Becker 1985; Becker and Maiman 1980; Chen 1991; Sackett and Haynes 1976). Although factors such as insight and motivation may render treatment adherence particularly challenging for psychiatric patients, the problem is not limited to the field of mental health. In fact, there have been reported similarly high rates of noncompliance with treatments for a large number of chronic medical conditions requiring long-term pharmacotherapy (Sackett and Haynes 1976). Most studies exploring correlates of noncompliance have focused on patient and treatment variables and have shown that a large number of factors significantly predict problems with adherence. These include patient sociodemographics, the financial burden associated with the treatment, and the side-effect profile of the medications (Fenton et al. 1997; Manne et al. 1993). The health-belief model has served as the theoretical framework for a large number of seminal research endeavors, which in aggregate demonstrate that the beliefs held by patients and those significant in their lives determine to a large extent their participation in and response to treatment decisions (Budd et al. 1996). The model has also been proven useful in guiding the development of intervention strategies that effectively enhance treatment adherence (Becker 1985; Haynes et al. 1987). In comparison, few empirical data are available on the influence of factors related to clinician(s) involved in the treatment, the site of treatment, and the nature and quality of the interactions between the clinician(s) and the patient (and those close to him or her).

Following the logic of the health-belief model, one would expect adherence to be an even larger problem in cross-cultural clinical situations. This has been substantiated by a number of clinical observations and reports of the use of services by particular ethnic minority groups (Sue et al. 1991). Compared with Caucasians, ethnic minority patients often enter treatment at a significantly delayed stage, and they also are more likely to drop out of psychiatric treatment prematurely. Programs aiming at bridging cultural gaps have been shown to improve treatment retention and outcome significantly (Acosta et al. 1982).

Findings from the following two studies underscore the importance of cultural factors in determining adherence to medication treatment: Kinzie et al. (1987) reported that 61% of their depressed, medicated refugee patients had no evidence of tricyclic antidepressants (TCAs) in their blood and that another 24% of them had only very low serum TCA levels, even though all of them were prescribed adequate TCA doses. When questioned, the patients admitted to being noncompliant for a variety of reasons. Education regarding the importance of long-term medication therapy and the maintenance of appropriate blood levels resulted in significant improvement in compliance in some but not all refugee groups. Similarly, in a study in South Africa (Gillis et al. 1987), 406 patients belonging to three ethnic groups (whites, blacks, and Asian Indians) were observed over a 2-year period after discharge from a psychiatric hospital. They found that approximately two-thirds of black patients, one-half of Asian Indian patients, and one-quarter of white patients were noncompliant with treatment with oral phenothiazines. The authors noted that the understanding of the treatment protocols by the relatives of the black and Asian Indian families was particularly poor, and culture and communication may have had significant effects on the results; however, one must also consider the impact of structural barriers such as cost and availability of transportation, as well as discrimination. Perhaps for analogous reasons, blacks in the United States are reportedly less compliant (D'Mello et al. 1989) and consequently are more likely to be prescribed injectable antipsychotics (Price et al. 1985).

Adverse effects of psychotropics are often substantial. Various drug-induced symptoms—including not only the classic extrapyramidal and anticholinergic side effects but also problems such as paradoxical agitation and weight gain—have been found to contribute significantly to noncompliance and treatment termination. Some of the most dramatic and disabling untoward effects of these therapeutic agents undoubtedly would be regarded with alarm by patients irrespective of their ethnic or cultural backgrounds (Glazer and Ereshefsky 1996). However, depending on patients' beliefs and expectations, many other drug effects could be interpreted as either negative or positive. For example, in a recent study of bipolar patients in Hong Kong who were treated with lithium, Lee et al. (1992) found that unlike Western patients, the Chinese rarely complained of "missing the highs" and "loss of creativity" and actually regarded polydipsia, polyuria, and weight gain as part of the therapeutic effect of the medicine. In contrast, lethargy, drowsiness, and poor memory were serious concerns for many of these patients and were prominent in their complaints, even though it was not likely that the conditions were due to the medication, given that they occurred at similar rates among matched control subjects. Such findings highlight the importance of culturally based beliefs and expectations in determining how physical and psychological experiences associated with drug treatment and recovery are attributed.

The explanatory model approach, as originally proposed by Kleinman (1988), may be a particularly effective way to assess such beliefs and expectations systematically. Methodically eliciting patients' perspectives on the symptoms that are most salient and worrisome to them (patterns of distress), their attributions (perceived causes), their help-seeking experiences and preferences, and their perceptions of stigma permits the discrepancy between patients' and professionals' explanatory models to be systematically identified and bridged (Weiss 1997). Currently being studied are the effectiveness and utility of such an approach with regard to enhancing treatment compliance, especially in terms of the use of psychotherapeutic agents, in various cultural settings. Elements of the explanatory model are also found in Appendix I of DSM-IV (American Psychiatric Association 1994), which includes an outline for cultural formulation. It is likely that the routine use of tools such as this will enable clinicians to improve adherence.

Expectation (Placebo) Effects

Although placebo control is an essential ingredient of modern clinical trials, the nature and determinants of the so-called placebo effect remain largely elusive and unexplored (Kleinman 1988; White et al. 1985). What is generally recognized, at least by researchers and administrators of regulatory agencies, is that such effects are typically substantial and often account for a larger proportion of the improvement than that attributable to the specific effect of the therapeutic agent being tested (Shepherd 1993; Swartzman and Burkell 1988). Despite the potency of the placebo, it has rarely been the primary focus of researchers' attention. Consequently, much ambiguity currently exists concerning this important phenomenon, and there is not even a consensus regarding which term to use when referring to such effects. The most commonly used term, *placebo,* carries a negative connotation and is easily misunderstood to imply deception as well as ineffectiveness. The term *nonspecific effect* could be similarly misleading, because many of the therapeutic effects elicited by "inert" agents might well be mediated through specific biological mechanisms (Weiner and Weiner 1996).

The concept of expectation effect, commonly used in psychotherapy research, may represent a broader and less controversial notion for such a phenomenon (Kirsch 1990; Tinsley et al. 1988). The term reflects the importance and power of expectation and beliefs concerning treatment effects in determining patient response to any therapy, whether psychosocial or pharmacological. Expectations regarding the safety and effectiveness of any therapeutic intervention, in turn, are shaped by patients' sociocultural backgrounds as well as individual experiences (e.g., past experiences of side effects). Given that patients' beliefs concerning medical treatments are often shaped by their cultural backgrounds, such cultural beliefs should potently determine patients' expectations regarding therapeutic effects of offered treatments.

Despite rapid modernization, traditional medical theories and practices remain deeply rooted and influential with regard to individuals' health beliefs and behaviors in many societies (Okpaku 1998; Rappaport 1977; Wig 1989; Wolffers 1989). For example, emphasized in most traditional medical systems is the importance of maintaining a dynamic balance between "coldness" and "hotness" (Castro et al. 1994) or between yin and yang, in the case of the Chinese system (Lin 1981). These principles provide guidance for assessment as well as for formulating treatment approaches. For patients who subscribe to such beliefs, a perceived mismatch between the therapeutic agents and the afflictions might significantly decrease the expectation effect. For example, red pills might be regarded as capable of enhancing the "hot" element and might be believed less effective in the treatment of conditions considered to be characterized by excessive "hotness" (e.g., fever, anxiety, or mania).

Buckalew and Coffield (1982) conducted a well-controlled study in which significant ethnic differences were found with regard to response to different-colored placebo pills. In this study, white capsules were seen as analgesics by Caucasian subjects but as stimulants by their African American counterparts. In contrast, black capsules were seen as stimulants by Caucasians and as analgesics by African Americans. Although the study did not specifically explore the symbolic meaning of these findings, the implications seem quite clear.

Concomitant Use of Modern and Alternative or Indigenous Treatments

As mentioned earlier, modern (Western) medicine has not eclipsed or replaced traditional or indigenous medical and healing systems (Engebretson and Wardell 1993; Frank 1974; Lin et al. 1990; Moerman 1979). Instead, alternative traditions (e.g., Chinese medicine and Ayurvedic medicine) seem to have responded well to challenges and have continued to evolve and thrive (Landy 1977; Leslie 1976). Thus, multiple medical and healing traditions and treatment modalities coexist in all societies, and patients often use these services simultaneously or sequentially, frequently without informing their physicians. Although this phenomenon has long been observed in non-Western countries (Kleinman 1988), as well as in ethnic minority populations in the United States (Chan and Chang 1976; "Leads from the MMWR"

1983; Vermeer and Ferrell 1985; Westermeyer 1989), its significance in Western societies probably has not been adequately appreciated until recent years. Thus, when Eisenberg et al. (1993) first reported that middle-class Americans (predominantly Caucasians) used more "alternative" medical services than outpatient "orthodox" medical care, the findings came as a surprise to most health care professionals. In the ensuing years, both in North America and Western Europe, there was an explosion in the popularity of a large number of alternative medical and healing methods, including many imported from non-Western traditions (Eisenberg et al. 1998; Wetzel et al. 1998). Thus, even though the concomitant use of alternative medicine and modern medicine may still be relatively more prevalent among ethnic minority populations, the problems that could arise from such a practice are no longer limited to particular groups but are of concern for all populations.

The efficacy of these alternative treatment methods and the validity of theories supporting the use of these interventions are subjects of frequent and rarely resolved debates, but there are what may be far more urgent and practical questions demanding even more immediate attention from researchers. Contrary to general perceptions, alternative treatments are not always mild or benign; some can induce severe toxic effects. Indeed, various herbs used by traditional practitioners and healers are biologically active. (It has been estimated that approximately 40% of modern pharmacotherapeutic agents originated from natural sources [Balick and Cox 1996]). Although much remains unclarified, what is beyond doubt is that herbal preparations often exert significant impact on various biological systems, including those crucial for the functioning of the central nervous system (Cott 1997; Duke 1995). For example, many herbal preparations have potent anticholinergic properties (Carbajal et al. 1991; Egashira et al. 1991; Yamahara et al. 1991) and may cause atropine psychosis, particularly when used concomitantly with psychotropics with similar side-effect profiles. Numerous herbs have distinctive stimulant or sedative properties and may either potentiate or attenuate the intended effects of medications prescribed by mental health practitioners (Amadi et al. 1991; Lewis et al. 1991). Because most patients do not regard herbs as medicines and typically fail to inform their physicians of use of herbs unless specifically asked, toxicities or treatment failures due to herb-drug interactions are likely widespread, of significant clinical consequence, but frequently unsuspected.

As will be elaborated later in this chapter and elsewhere in this volume, a limited number of enzymes are involved in the biotransformation of all drugs, including psychotropics. Although the activity of these enzymes is crucial for determining the pharmacokinetics and hence the fate and disposition of modern drugs, their primary targets are not the medications prescribed by physicians but xenobiotics (natural substances) existing in the organisms' environments that are potentially toxic (Gonzalez and Nebert 1990). Many herbs are thus natural substrates for these drug-metabolizing enzymes. Further, through inhibition and/or induction, xenobiotics, including a large number of herbs (Liu 1991), exert powerful influences on the expression of these enzymes, which then determines the rate of metabolism of the medications prescribed. Thus, herbal medicines may modulate the effect of modern therapeutic agents, including psychotropics, not only at the pharmacodynamic level (the effect of the drugs on the organism) but also at the pharmacokinetic level.

Biological Diversity and Psychotropic Responses

The central importance of biodiversity in maintaining and ensuring the survival of any species and promoting its adaptation to the local environment is a fundamental principle that often has not been adequately appreciated (Hughes et al. 1997; Marwick 1995). Possibly because of the underappreciation of the extent and significance of biological diversity in the past, recent findings of the widespread existence of genetic polymorphisms have appeared surprising to many researchers. However, emerging data now convincingly demonstrate that for the majority of the genes, polymorphism is the rule rather than the exception. Furthermore, the frequency and distribution of alleles responsible for such polymorphisms often vary substantially across ethnic groups, and

Table 1–1. Genetically variable enzymes of drug metabolism

N-Acetyltransferase[a]	Dihydropyrimidine dehydrogenase
Alcohol dehydrogenase[a]	Dopamine β-hydroxylase
Aldehyde dehydrogenase[a]	Glucuronyl transferase[a]
Butyryl cholinesterase	Glutathione S-transferase (class μ)[a]
Catalase	Monoamine oxidase
Catechol O-methyltransferase[a]	Phenol sulfotransferase[a]
CYP1A2[a]	Serum paroxanase/arylesterase[a]
CYP2A6[a]	Superoxide dismutase
CYP2C19[a]	Thiol methyltransferase[a]
CYP2D6[a]	Thiopurine methyltransferase[a]
CYP2E1[a]	
CYP3A4[a]	

[a]Polymorphic variation.
Source. Adapted from Kalow 1992 and Lin and Poland 1995.

therefore ethnicity should always be considered in genetic studies (National Institute of Mental Health 1999). These phenomena have long been recognized in blood and human lymphocyte antigen typing (Polednak 1989). In recent years, it has become increasingly clear that equally extensive polymorphisms exist in genes governing key aspects of how drugs are metabolized (see Table 1–1) as well as how they affect the target organs. These processes, commonly called *pharmacokinetics* and *pharmacodynamics,* are depicted in Figure 1–2 (Greenblatt 1993). Together, these genetic factors may explain to a large extent the often extensive interindividual cross-ethnic variations in drug responses (Kalow 1992; Lin et al. 1993). In the following sections, some of the relevant findings in these regards are highlighted.

Genetic Polymorphism of Genes Encoding Drug-Metabolizing Enzymes

As shown in Figure 1–2, of the four factors (absorption, distribution, metabolism, and excretion) that together determine the fate and disposition of most drugs, variability in metabolism is most substantial and usually is the reason for interindividual and cross-ethnic variations in drug responses (Lin and Poland 1995). Most drugs are metabolized in two phases. Phase I, commonly mediated by one or more of the cytochrome P450 (CYP) enzymes, leads

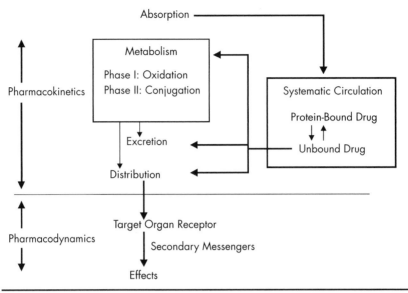

Figure 1–2.   Pharmacokinetics and pharmacodynamics.

to the oxidation of the substrate; phase II involves conjugation and is usually mediated by one of the transferases. There is clear evidence of interindividual and cross-ethnic variations in the activity of the enzymes in both phases, the genetic basis of which has been increasingly elucidated in recent years (Kalow 1992; Weber 1997). Because far more information is currently available regarding the CYPs than the phase II enzymes, and because the CYPs appear to control the rate-limiting steps in the metabolism of most psychotropics, the main focus of the following discussion is on these enzymes.

Table 1–2 includes a list of major CYPs that are responsible for the phase I metabolism of commonly used psychotropics as well as selected substances that are psychoactive and are commonly used by psychiatric patients. With very few exceptions (e.g., lithium does not require biotransformation; lorazepam and oxazepam are directly conjugated without first going through oxidation), the pharmacokinetics of practically all psychotropics are dependent on one or more of the CYPs, whose activity significantly influences the tissue concentrations, dose requirement, and side-effect profiles of their substrates.

Table 1–2. Major human cytochrome P450 enzymes and their psychotropic substrates

Enzyme[a]	Substrates	Genetic polymorphisms
CYP1A2	*Antidepressants:* amitriptyline, clomipramine, imipramine, fluvoxamine *Neuroleptics:* haloperidol, phenothiazines, thiothixene, clozapine, olanzapine *Others:* tacrine, caffeine, theophylline, acetaminophen, phenacetin	No report of polymorphism until 1999; significance of following findings remains unclear: *1C: reduced activity; 23% in Japanese *1F: higher inducibility; 32% in Caucasians
CYP2C19	*Benzodiazepines:* diazepam *Antidepressants:* imipramine, amitriptyline, clomipramine, citalopram *Others:* propranolol, hexobarbital, mephobarbital, proguanil, omeprazole, S-mephenytoin	*2: no activity; 23%–39% in Asians; 13% in Caucasians; 25% in African Americans *3: no activity; 6%–10% in Asians; 0% in others
CYP2D6	*Antidepressants:* amitriptyline, clomipramine, imipramine, desipramine, nortriptyline, trimipramine, N-desmethyl-clomipramine, fluoxetine, norfluoxetine, paroxetine, venlafaxine, sertraline *Neuroleptics:* chlorpromazine, thioridazine, perphenazine, haloperidol, reduced haloperidol, risperidone, clozapine, sertindole *Others:* codeine, opiate, propranolol, dextromethorphan	*4: no activity; 25% in Caucasians; 0%–10% in others *5: no activity; 2%–10% in all groups *10: reduced activity; 47%–70% in Asians; ≤5% in others *17: reduced activity; 25%–40% in blacks; 0% in others *2XN: increased activity; 19%–29% in Arabs and Ethiopians; ≤5% in others

Table 1–2. Major human cytochrome P450 enzymes and their psychotropic substrates *(continued)*

Enzyme[a]	Substrates	Genetic polymorphisms
CYP3A4	*Antidepressants:* mirtazapine, nefazodone, sertraline *Neuroleptics:* thioridazine, haloperidol, clozapine, quetiapine, risperidone, sertindole, ziprasidone *Mood stabilizers:* carbamazepine, gabapentin, lamotrigine *Benzodiazepines:* alprazolam, clonazepam, diazepam, midazolam, triazolam, zolpidem *Calcium channel blockers:* diltiazem, nifedipine, nimodipine, verapamil *Steroids:* androgens, estrogens, cortisol *Others:* erythromycin, terfenadine, cyclosporine, dapsone, ketoconazole, lovastatin, lidocaine, alfentanil, amiodarone, astemizole, codeine, sildenafil	No clear evidence of polymorphism; recent reports of functional significance of variant with mutation in regulatory region (*1B) disputed; prevalence of *1B is 10% in Caucasians and unknown in other ethnic groups; preliminary reports of two other promising alleles (*2 and *3), but details of these mutations not yet available

[a]Other important human cytochrome P450 enzymes include CYP2A6, CYP2B6, CYP2C8, CYP2C9, and CYP2E1. CYP2A6 is involved in the metabolism of nicotine and cotinine; CYP2C9 is responsible for the biotransformation of drugs, including phenytoin and warfarin; and CYP2E1 metabolizes acetaminophen and theophylline, as well as alcohol, and is associated with the production of free radicals.

Functionally significant genetic polymorphisms exist in most of the CYPs (Lin and Poland 1995), leading to extremely large variations in the activity of these enzymes in any given population. CYP2D6 is the most dramatic example, with more than 20 mutations that inactivate, impair, or accelerate its function (Daly et al. 1996). Significantly, most of these mutant alleles are, to a large extent, ethnically specific. For example, *CYP2D6*4 (CYP2D6B)*, which leads to the production of defective proteins, is found in approximately 25% of Caucasians but is rarely identified in other ethnic groups. This mutation is mainly responsible for the high percentage of poor metabolizers (PMs) among Caucasians (5%–9%), who are extremely sensitive to drugs metabolized by CYP2D6 (see Figure 1–3). Instead of *CYP2D6*4*, extremely high frequencies of *CYP2D6*17* (Leathart et al. 1998; Masimirembwa and Hasler 1997) and *CYP2D6*10* (Dahl et al. 1995; Roh et al. 1996; Wang et al. 1993) were found among those of African and Asian origins, respectively. Both of these alleles are associated with lower enzyme activities and slower metabolism of CYP2D6 substrates (Figure 1–3) and may be responsible in part for previous findings of slower pharmacokinetic profiles and lower dose ranges observed in Asians, with regard to both classes of psychotropics, and in African Americans, with regard to TCAs (Lin and Poland 1995). Our recent study showed that Mexican Americans had very low rates of any of these "impairing" mutations. Correspondingly, they also showed evidence of significantly faster overall CYP2D6 activity (Mendoza et al., submitted).

CYP2D6 also is unique in that the gene often is duplicated or multiplied (up to 13 copies). Individuals possessing these duplicated or multiple genes have proportionally more enzymes and faster enzyme activity and are termed *superextensive metabolizers.* This phenomenon is found in 1% of Swedes, 5% of Spaniards (the percentage of white Americans who are superextensive metabolizers is between these two figures), 19% of Arabs, and 29% of Ethiopians. Superextensive metabolizers are likely to fail to respond to usual doses of medications biotransformed by CYP2D6; they typically require extremely high doses of these drugs to achieve therapeutic levels. There have been reports of superextensive metabolizers' being regarded as noncompliant because

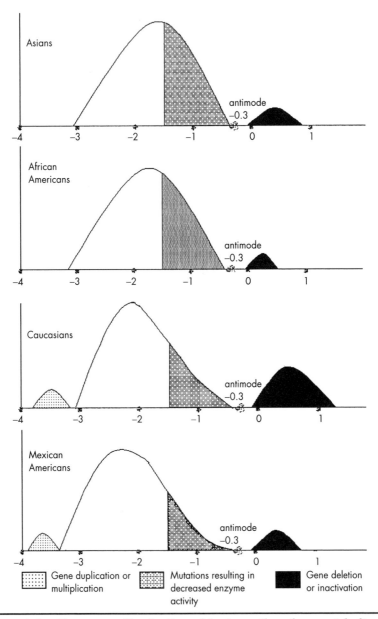

Figure 1–3. Frequency distribution of dextromethorphan metabolic ratios (MRs) in Asians, African Americans, Caucasians, and Mexican Americans. The MR is the $\log_{10}$ of the ratio between urinary dextromethorphan and one of its main metabolites, dextrophan. Lower MRs indicate more active enzyme activities.

they did not show any evidence of drug effect when given seemingly adequate doses of medications (Aklillu et al. 1996).

CYP2C19 provides more evidence of the existence of both cross-ethnic and interindividual variations in drug metabolism. This enzyme is involved in the metabolism of commonly used psychotropics such as diazepam and tertiary TCAs, as well as one of the new antidepressants, citalopram. Using S-mephenytoin as the probe, earlier studies demonstrated that up to 20% of East Asians (Chinese, Japanese, and Koreans) are PMs, compared with only 3%–5% of Caucasians. After the gene for the enzyme had been identified and sequenced, it became clear that such enzyme deficiency is caused by two unique mutations (CYP2C19*2 and CYP2C19*3). Whereas *2 can be found in all ethnic groups, *3 appears to be specific to those of East Asian origin. The presence of *3, together with a higher rate of *2, is responsible for the higher percentage of PMs among Asians, as well as their often increased sensitivity to drugs such as diazepam (de Morais et al. 1994; Goldstein et al. 1997).

Genetic polymorphism also exists in CYP1A2, CYP2C9, CYP2E1, CYP3A4, and the majority of other drug-metabolizing enzymes (see Tables 1–1 and 1–2). It is interesting to note that, almost without exception, wherever genetic polymorphism is identified, the allele frequency of mutations typically varies substantially across ethnic groups (Gill et al. 1999; Kidd et al. 1999; Stephens et al. 1994).

Factors Affecting Expression of Drug-Metabolizing Enzymes

In addition to genetic endowment, a large number of nongenetic factors also significantly influence the expression of the genes. These factors are both external and internal. External factors include nutrients, various plant products, pharmaceutical agents, and other chemicals. Internal factors include steroid hormones and other endogenous substances (Anderson et al. 1987; Bolt 1994). These substances either inhibit or induce the activity of the enzyme and thus affect the metabolism of drugs that are dependent on a particular enzyme. Such shifts in the enzyme status could at times lead to serious clinical consequences.

The following are selected examples from recent years: 1) A number of the newer antidepressants—including fluoxetine and paroxetine, two of the most widely used selective serotonin reuptake inhibitors (SSRIs)—are potent inhibitors of CYP2D6, capable of converting an extensive metabolizer into a PM. Thus, when one of these drugs is prescribed to a patient who has already been taking a CYP2D6 substrate (e.g., a TCA or a neuroleptic), the concentration of the substrate could be pushed unexpectedly into the toxic range (Aranow et al. 1989; Bergstrom et al. 1992; Brosen 1995). 2) Smoking has long been known to reduce the serum concentration of psychotropics significantly, and it is likely that many patients relapse soon after discharge from the hospital because they resume smoking (Guengerich et al. 1994). This effect is now known to be due to the induction of CYP1A2 by constituents of tobacco (DeVane 1994). 3) Many drugs and natural substances significantly inhibit the activity of CYP3A4, altering its ability to metabolize drugs that are dependent on this enzyme for their biotransformation. A widely known example is grapefruit juice (Fuhr et al. 1993; Oesterheld and Kallepalli 1997), which is capable of increasing severalfold the blood level of antiviral drugs as well as psychotropics such as nefazodone and alprazolam, if the juice and one of these drugs are taken concurrently. In addition, reports of death caused by the combination of ketoconazole and terfenadine have led to the withdrawal of the latter from the market (Jurima-Romet et al. 1994). 4) A large body of literature indicates that high-protein and high-carbohydrate diets also significantly influence the activity of CYP enzymes. A high-protein diet accelerates the metabolism of drugs such as antipyrine and theophylline, and a high-carbohydrate diet appears to have the opposite effect (Anderson and Kappas 1991; Branch et al. 1978; Fraser et al. 1979).

These examples demonstrate that environmental factors substantially modify the activity of these drug-metabolizing enzymes. Patients from different ethnic or cultural backgrounds have divergent lifestyles and likely are exposed to unique substances that may have strong effects on the expression and activity of drug-metabolizing enzymes. Thus, what is currently known about environmental influences on drug metabolism may represent only the tip of the iceberg. This may be especially true in regard to ethnic minority and other non-Western populations. For example, studies have shown that Asian Indians and Africans were significantly slower in metabolizing substrates of CYP1A2, such as theophylline, antipyrine, and clomipramine. However, after they immigrated to Europe and adopted the new dietary habits, their metabolic profiles for these drugs became indistinguishable from native Westerners' (Allen et al. 1977).

As discussed earlier, herbal medicines are routinely and extensively used by people worldwide, and there are theoretical bases, supported by empirical data, for believing that many herbs significantly modify the expression of drug-metabolizing enzymes by either inhibition or induction (Liu 1991). Because patients typically are not aware of the potential of herb-drug interactions, they often combine the use of herbs with the use of Western medicines. When severe toxic effects subsequently occur, they usually blame them on drugs prescribed by clinicians, rather than on herbal preparations obtained over the counter or from practitioners of traditional or alternative medicine (Smith et al. 1993). Because thousands of herbs are in wide use, and the indication and popularity of these herbs vary a great deal across cultural traditions, the potential for interactions between herbs and modern pharmaceutical agents is endless and largely unexplored (Smith et al. 1993).

Genetic Polymorphism of Genes Encoding Receptors, Transporters, or Other Therapeutic Targets

Monoamines, including dopamine, serotonin, and norepinephrine, have been the focus of intensive research during the past several decades. In addition to being implicated in the pathogenesis of psychiatric disorders, including schizophrenia and major depression, they have also been regarded as the putative targets of psychotropics (Barker and Blakely 1996). Confirming the importance of the serotonin system in affective and other psychiatric disorders is the fact that a number of SSRIs have been developed and are now in use for a wide range of clinical conditions. At the same time, although the far more diffuse receptor-binding profiles of the atypical neuroleptics call into question the primacy of the "dopamine hypothesis" in schizophrenia research, the function of the dopaminergic system remains important in understanding the schizophrenic process and its pharmacological management (Bloom et al. 1995).

In addition to the cloning and sequencing of the genes encoding the receptors and transporters that mediate and regulate the function of these important neurotransmitters, it has become apparent that, contrary to earlier predictions (Kalow 1990), these genes are almost without exception highly polymorphic, and the pattern of these polymorphisms varies significantly across ethnicity (Chang et al. 1996; Dean et al. 1994; Gelenter et al. 1997; Goldman et al. 1996; Hodge 1994). For example, the frequency of the *Taq*I A RFLP polymorphism of the D_2 dopamine receptor *(DRD2)*, one of the most extensively investigated brain receptors, ranges from 5% to 18% in Caucasians to approximately 36% in African Americans and 37%–42% in Asians (Blum et al. 1995). Earlier studies suggesting the existence of an association between this allele and alcoholism have been criticized because ethnicity was not taken into consideration as a potential confounding variable. Similarly dramatic ethnic variations exist in the pattern of genetic polymorphism of many other receptor and transporter genes. These include other *DRD2* mutations *(Taq1* B, 311Ser/Cys, and exon 8 A/G substitution), other dopamine receptors such as *DRD4* and *DRD3* (Parsian et al. 1997; Sander et al. 1995; Sullivan et al. 1998), the dopamine transporter gene *(DAT1*; locus symbol SLC6A3) (Vandenbergh et al. 1992), the serotonin transporter gene *(5-HTT)*, and a number of serotonin receptors *(5HT2A-1438 A/G* and *5HT2A-102 T/C)* (Greenberg et al. 1998; Michaelovsky et al. 1999; Smeraldi et al. 1998).

These polymorphisms likely have functional significance and hence might be associated with the risk of psychopathology as well as response to treatment regimens. For example, recent studies show that the basal transcriptional activity of *5-HTT* is significantly higher in those possessing a long variant in the promoter region of this gene, which results in differential *5-HTT* expression and 5-HT cellular uptake (Greenberg et al. 1998). The clinical significance of these findings was recently demonstrated in a study of the effect of treatment with SSRIs on psychotic depression (Smeraldi et al. 1998). In this study, patients who were either homozygote or heterozygote long variant (*5-HTTLPR l/l* and *l/s*) responded significantly better than those who were homozygote short variant (*s/s*). Similarly, *DRD2 Taq*I A RFLP polymorphism, located in the 3' flanking region of the *DRD2* gene, has been shown in brain imaging (Hietala et al. 1994) and postmortem (Noble et al. 1991) studies to affect D_2 receptor density in different parts of the brain, and thus the polymorphism might affect the receptor's response to neuroleptics, in addition to its possible association with the risk of alcoholism. However, it is unclear whether such associations exist across ethnic groups and whether ethnic differences in the polymorphisms might result in ethnic variations in the pharmacodynamics of drugs whose effects are mediated by these receptors or transporters.

Genetic Polymorphism of Other Genes Affecting Pharmacological Responses

The synthesis and catabolism of the catecholamines are controlled by a number of enzymes, including tryptophan hydroxylase, tyrosine hydroxylase, catechol *O*-methyltransferase (COMT), and the monoamine oxidases (MAOs). Tryptophan hydroxylase controls the rate-limiting step for the production of serotonin from tryptophan (Smeraldi et al. 1998), and tyrosine hydroxylase plays a central role in the production of dopamine and norepinephrine. On the catabolic side, MAO mediates the oxidation and deamination of serotonin into 5-hydroxyindoleacetic acid (5-HIAA) and other metabolites, and both MAO and COMT are responsible for the metabolism of the catecholamines (dopamine and norepinephrine). Interestingly, all of these enzymes are highly polymorphic (Jonsson et al. 1997). For example, COMT activity has long been known to have a trimodal distribution (Li et al. 1997; McLeod et al. 1994). Recent studies demonstrate that the reduction of its activity is caused by a single nucleotide mutation whose allele frequency is approximately 26% in African Americans, 18% in Asians, and 50% in Caucasians (de Chaldee et al. 1999; Daniels et al. 1996). Higher COMT activity is correlated with the ratio between 3-*O*-methyldopa and levodopa, which in turn predicts the occurrence of side effects of levodopa in treating parkinsonism.

Reflecting this, a higher percentage of Asians have been found to be poor responders to levodopa (Rivera-Calimlim and Reilly 1984). It is at present unclear whether such interindividual and cross-ethnic variations in the polymorphism of these enzymes influence the pharmacodynamics of psychotropics used in clinical settings.

It is commonly agreed that the signal transduction cascade, which is much less understood, is also of tremendous importance in mediating the effect of psychotropics. Components of this cascade include G proteins, ion channels, second messengers, and protein kinases (Manji et al. 1995). Interindividual and cross-ethnic variations in the genes coding these proteins likely exist and may also be responsible for the individual variability in drug response observed clinically.

Summary and Future Research Directions

This brief survey serves to highlight the significance as well as the complexity of issues surrounding the influence of cultural and ethnic forces on psychotropic responses. Taken together, the literature reviewed here clearly demonstrates the importance of these factors in practicing psychopharmacotherapy. At the same time, it is equally important that any findings regarding ethnic variations in pharmacological responses not be interpreted stereotypically. In this regard, it is useful to keep in mind that almost all ethnic and cultural contrasts are superimposed on usually very substantial interindividual variations in all human groups. (For an example of this, see Figure 1–4.) This is true not only with regard to biological traits such as the ones just reviewed, but equally so (or even more so) with regard to cultural and psychosocial variables. Stereotypical interpretations of cultural and ethnic differences in either psychological or biological characteristics are not only misleading but also potentially divisive and dangerous.

Further, in interpreting biological diversity, both within and across populations, it is important to keep in mind that biological systems are dynamic rather than static and the expression of genetic predisposition is constantly modified by environmental exposure. This is most clearly demonstrated in the case of the

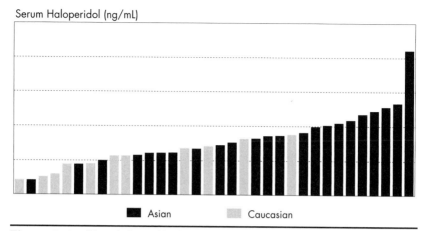

Serum Haloperidol (ng/mL)

■ Asian   ▦ Caucasian

Figure 1–4. Variability of haloperidol concentrations in psychiatrically healthy volunteers after intramuscular injection of 0.5 mg haloperidol. The graph shows substantial interindividual variability within each ethnic group, dramatic differences in the pharmacokinetics of haloperidol between the two groups, and overlap of the pharmacokinetics between the two groups.
Source. Reprinted from Lin K-M, Poland RE, Lau JK, et al.: "Haloperidol and Prolactin Concentrations in Asians and Caucasians." *J Clin Psychopharmacol* 8:195–201, 1988. Used with permission.

induction and inhibition of the drug-metabolizing enzymes, which could radically alter an individual's metabolic profile, such that a genetic extensive metabolizer might appear to possess nonfunctioning gene(s). Although it is reasonable to believe that social and psychological events would similarly exert powerful influences on the functioning of relevant genes, such influences are likely to be far more subtle and complex and have remained largely unexplored.

In addition to culture and ethnicity, other key sociodemographic variables, such as age and sex, have also been known to influence significantly the pharmacokinetics and pharmacodynamics of psychotropics and other pharmaceutical agents (Jensvold et al. 1996). For example, the activity of most P450 enzymes declines substantially in older individuals (Kinirons and Crome 1997; Tanaka 1998), who are also likely to have progressive loss of neuron cells as well as receptors targeted by psychotropics (Salzman

1984). Both of these changes render elderly persons more sensitive to the effects of medications in general. Similarly, steroid hormones including sex hormones have been demonstrated to be substrates of some of the P450 enzymes and have the capacity to alter the activity of these enzymes through competitive inhibition and/or other mechanisms. They also have been known to exert powerful influences on some of the brain receptors that might directly or indirectly affect the pharmacodynamics of psychotropics (Jensvold et al. 1996). It is unclear at present to what extent such age and sex effects interact with the effect of ethnicity and whether such interactions are synergistic or additive. Studies examining such interactions might be of utmost clinical importance, because they might help to identify groups with heightened possibility of unusual dose response and side-effect profiles.

Progress in the research on P450 enzymes and other drug-metabolizing enzymes in the past three decades has led to the development of a number of laboratory procedures that could be used for determining the activity of these enzymes as well as polymorphisms of the genes encoding them. These procedures have been found to be predictive of the pharmacokinetics and side-effect profiles of a number of psychotropics. In addition, emergent data suggest that some of the polymorphisms of genes encoding neurotransmitter transporters and/or receptors might also predict treatment outcome. Thus, it appears that technology may be in place for researchers to test the utility of these procedures systematically in clinical settings. It is likely that progress in this direction will eventually lead to the development of a panel of genotyping and/or phenotyping procedures that could be used by clinicians to guide their decisions in terms of the choice of antidepressants, starting doses, and strategies for titration, as well to predict likely side effects. Such a panel will not only enhance the treatment response rate but also reduce the duration of dose titration and minimize the development of untoward effects and therefore ensure better treatment compliance. Thus, it should also result in treatment strategies that are both more effective and more cost-effective than traditional titration methods. With the development of high-throughput gene array technologies (Hacia et al. 1998), such as matrix-assisted laser desorption/ionization time-of-flight mass spectroscopy (Ross et al. 1998), thousands of samples could be processed on a daily basis, so that the turnaround time for test results could be short enough to be useful for clinicians ordering such tests. Together, these exciting new developments should help to make psychopharmacotherapy increasingly more rational, evidence based, and effective.

The progress in pharmacogenetics might also stimulate research into nonbiological issues such as cultural influences on adherence and other factors that determine patients' perceptions and actions, which in turn contribute to their sense of satisfaction and their ability to obtain maximum benefit from antidepressant treatment. With such an integrative approach, physicians would be best able to define elements for optimal pharmacotherapeutic practices that would take both cultural and biological diversity into consideration and tailor treatment to individual characteristics rather than rely on global guidelines.

References

Acosta FX, Yamamoto J, Evans LA: Effective Psychotherapy for Low-Income and Minority Patients. New York, Plenum, 1982

Adebimpe VR: Overview: white norms and psychiatric diagnosis of black patients. Am J Psychiatry 138:279–285, 1981

Aklillu E, Persson I, Bertilsson L, et al: Frequent distribution of ultrarapid metabolizers of debrisoquine in an Ethiopian population carrying duplicated and multiduplicated functional CYP2D6 alleles. J Pharmacol Exp Ther 278:441–446, 1996

Allen JG, Rack P, Vaddadi K: Differences in the effects of clomipramine on English and Asian volunteers: preliminary report on a pilot study. Postgrad Med J 53:79–86, 1977

Amadi E, Offiah N, Akah P: Neuropsychopharmacologic properties of a *Schumanniophyton problematicum* root extract. J Ethnopharmacol 33:73–77, 1991

American Psychiatric Association: Diagnostic and Statistical Manual of Mental Disorders, 4th Edition. Washington, DC, American Psychiatric Association, 1994

Anderson KE, Kappas A: Dietary regulation of cytochrome P450. Annu Rev Nutr 11:141–167, 1991

Anderson KE, Rosner W, Khan MS, et al: Diet-hormone interactions: protein/carbohydrate ratio alters reciprocally the plasma levels of testosterone and cortisol and their respective binding globulins in man. Life Sci 40:1761–1768, 1987

Aranow RB, Hudson JI, Pope HG, et al: Elevated antidepressant plasma levels after addition of fluoxetine. Am J Psychiatry 146:911–913, 1989

Balick MJ, Cox PA: Plants, People, and Culture: The Science of Ethnobotany. New York, Scientific American Library, 1996

Barker EL, Blakely RD: Identification of a single amino acid, phenylalanine 586, that is responsible for high affinity interactions of tricyclic antidepressants with the human serotonin transporter. Molecular Pharmacology 50(4):957–965, 1996

Becker MH: Patient adherence to prescribed therapies. Med Care 23:539–555, 1985

Becker MH, Maiman LA: Strategies for enhancing patient compliance. J Community Health 6:113–135, 1980

Bergstrom RF, Peyton AL, Lemberger L: Quantification and mechanism of the fluoxetine and tricyclic antidepressant interaction. Clin Pharmacol Ther 51:239–248, 1992

Bloom FE, Kupfer D: Psychopharmacology: The Fourth Generation of Progress. New York, Raven, 1995

Blum K, Sheridan PJ, Wood RC, et al: Dopamine D2 receptor gene variants: association and linkage studies in impulsive-addictive-compulsive behaviour. Pharmacogenetics 5(3):121–141, 1995

Bolt HM: Interactions between clinically used drugs and oral contraceptives. Environ Health Perspect 102 (suppl 9):35–38, 1994

Branch RA, Salih SY, Homeida M: Racial differences in drug metabolizing ability: a study with antipyrine in the Sudan. Clin Pharmacol Ther 24:283–286, 1978

Brosen K: Drug interactions and the cytochrome P450 system. Clin Pharmacokinet 29:20–25, 1995

Buckalew LW, Coffield K: Drug expectations associated with perceptual characteristics: ethnic factors. Percept Mot Skills 55:915–918, 1982

Budd RJ, Hughes IC, Smith JA: Health beliefs and compliance with antipsychotic medication. Br J Clin Psychol 35(3):393–397, 1996

Carbajal D, Casaco A, Arruzazabala L: Pharmacological screening of plant decoctions commonly used in Cuban folk medicine. J Ethnopharmacol 33:21–24, 1991

Castro FG, Furth P, Karlow H: The health beliefs of Mexican, Mexican-American and Anglo-American women. Hispanic Journal of Behavioral Sciences 6:365–383, 1994

Chan CW, Chang JK: The role of Chinese medicine in New York City's Chinatown. Am J Chin Med 4:31–45, 129–146, 1976

Chang FM, Kidd JR, Livak KJ, et al: The world-wide distribution of allele frequencies at the human dopamine D4 receptor locus. Hum Genet 98:91–101, 1996

Chen A: Noncompliance in community psychiatry: a review of clinical interventions. Hospital and Community Psychiatry 42:282–287, 1991

Cott JM: In vitro receptor binding and enzyme inhibition by *Hypericum perforatum* extract. Pharmacopsychiatry 30 (suppl 2):108–112, 1997

Dahl ML, Yue QY, Roh HK, et al: Genetic analysis of the CYP2D locus in relation to debrisoquine hydroxylation capacity in Korean, Japanese and Chinese subjects. Pharmacogenetics 5:159–164, 1995

Daly AK, Brockmoller J, Broly F, et al: Nomenclature for human CYP2D6 alleles. Pharmacogenetics 6:193–201, 1996

Daniels JK, Williams NM, Williams J, et al: No evidence for allelic association between schizophrenia and a polymorphism determining high or low catechol O-methyltransferase activity. Am J Psychiatry 153(2):268–270, 1996

Dean M, Stephens JC, Winkler C, et al: Polymorphic admixture typing in human ethnic populations. Am J Hum Genet 55:788–808, 1994

de Chaldee M, Laurent C, Thibaut F, et al: Linkage disequilibrium on the COMT gene in French schizophrenics and controls. Am J Med Genet 88(5):452–457, 1999

de Morais SM, Wilkinson GR, Blaisdell J, et al: The major genetic defect responsible for the polymorphism of *S*-mephenytoin metabolism in humans. J Biol Chem 269:15419–15422, 1994

DeVane CL: Pharmacogenetics and drug metabolism of newer antidepressant agents. J Clin Psychiatry 55 (suppl):38–45, 1994

D'Mello DA, McNeil JA, Harris W: Multi-ethnic variance in psychiatric diagnosis and neuroleptic dosage. Paper presented at the annual meeting of the American Psychiatric Association, San Francisco, CA, May 6–11, 1989

Duke JA: Commentary—novel psychotherapeutic drugs: a role for ethnobotany. Psychopharmacol Bull 31:177–184, 1995

Egashira T, Sudo S, Murayama F, et al: Effects of kamikihi-to, a Chinese traditional medicine, on various cholinergic biochemical markers in the brains of aged rats [in Japanese]. Nippon Yakurigaku Zasshi 98:273–281, 1991

Eisenberg DM, Kessler RC, Foster C, et al: Unconventional medicine in the United States: prevalence, cost, and patterns of use. N Engl J Med 328:246–252, 1993

Eisenberg DM, Davis RB, Ettner SL, et al: Trends in alternative medicine use in the United States, 1990–1997: results of a follow-up national survey. JAMA 280:1569–1575, 1998

Engebretson J, Wardell D: A contemporary view of alternative healing modalities. Nurse Pract 18:51–55, 1993

Fenton WS, Blyler CR, Heinssen RK: Determinants of medication compliance in schizophrenia: empirical and clinical findings. Schizophr Bull 23:637–651, 1997

Frank JD: Persuasion and Healing: A Comparative Study of Psychotherapy. New York, Schocken Books, 1974

Fraser HS, Mucklow JC, Bulpitt CJ, et al: Environmental factors affecting antipyrine metabolism in London factory and office workers. Br J Clin Pharmacol 7:237–243, 1979

Fuhr U, Klittich K, Staib AH: Inhibitory effect of grapefruit juice and its bitter principal, naringenin, on CYP1A2 dependent metabolism of caffeine in man. Br J Clin Pharmacol 35:431–436, 1993

Gaw A: Culture, Ethnicity, and Mental Illness. Washington, DC, American Psychiatric Press, 1993

Gelenter J, Kranzler H, Cubells JF, et al: Serotonin transporter protein (SLC6A4) allele and haplotype frequencies and linkage disequilibria in African- and European-American and Japanese populations and in alcohol-dependent subjects. Hum Genet 101:243–246, 1997

Gill HJ, Tjia JF, Kitteringham NR, et al: The effect of genetic polymorphisms in CYP2C9 on sulphamethoxazole N-hydroxylation. Pharmacogenetics 9:43–53, 1999

Gillis L, Trollip D, Jakoet A, et al: Non-compliance with psychotropic medication. S Afr Med J 72:602–606, 1987

Glazer WM, Ereshefsky L: A pharmacoeconomic model of outpatient antipsychotic therapy in "revolving door" schizophrenic patients. J Clin Psychiatry 57:337–345, 1996

Goldman D, Lappalainen J, Ozaki N: Direct analysis of candidate genes in impulsive behaviours. Ciba Found Symp 194:139–152, 1996

Goldstein JA, Ishizaki T, Chiba K, et al: Frequencies of the defective CYP2C19 alleles responsible for the mephenytoin poor metabolizer phenotype in various Oriental, Caucasian, Saudi Arabian and American black populations. Pharmacogenetics 7:59–64, 1997

Gonzalez FJ, Nebert DW: Evolution of the P450 gene superfamily: animal-plant 'warfare,' molecular drive and human genetic differences in drug oxidation. Trends Genet 6:182–186, 1990

Greenberg BD, McMahon FJ, Murphy DL: Serotonin transporter candidate gene studies in affective disorders and personality: promises and potential pitfalls. Mol Psychiatry 3:186–189, 1998

Greenblatt DJ: Basic pharmacokinetic principles and their application to psychotropic drugs. J Clin Psychiatry 54:8–13, 1993

Guengerich FP, Shimada T, Yun CH, et al: Interactions of ingested food, beverage, and tobacco components involving human cytochrome P4501A2, 2A6, 2E1, and 3A4 enzymes. Environ Health Perspect 102 (suppl 9):49–53, 1994

Hacia JG, Brody LC, Collins FS: Applications of DNA chips for genomic analysis. Mol Psychiatry 3:483–492, 1998

Haynes R, Wang E, da Mota Gomez M: A critical review of interventions to improve compliance with prescribed medications. Patient Educ Couns 10:155–166, 1987

Hietala J, West C, Syvalahti E, et al: Striatal D2 dopamine receptor binding characteristics in vivo in patients with alcohol dependence. Psychopharmacology 116:285–290, 1994

Hodge SE: What association analysis can and cannot tell us about the genetics of complex disease. Am J Med Genet 54:318–323, 1994

Hughes JB, Daily GC, Ehrlich PR: Population diversity: its extent and extinction. Science 278:689–692, 1997

Jensvold MF, Halbreich U, Hamilton JA: Psychopharmacology and Women: Sex, Gender, and Hormones. Washington, DC, American Psychiatric Press, 1996, 121–136

Jonsson EG, Goldman D, Spurlock G, et al: Tryptophan hydroxylase and catechol-O-methyltransferase gene polymorphisms: relationships to monoamine metabolite concentrations in CSF of healthy volunteers. Eur Arch Psychiatry Clin Neurosci 247:297–302, 1997

Jurima-Romet M, Crawford K, Cyr T, et al: Terfenadine metabolism in human liver: in vitro inhibition by macrolide antibiotics and azole antifungals. Drug Metab Dispos 22:849–857, 1994

Kalow W: Pharmacogenetics: past and future. Life Sci 47:1385–1397, 1990

Kalow W: Pharmacogenetics of Drug Metabolism. New York, Pergamon, 1992

Kidd RS, Straughn AB, Meyer MC, et al: Pharmacokinetics of chlorpheniramine, phenytoin, glipizide and nifedipine in an individual homozygous for the CYP2C9*3 allele. Pharmacogenetics 9:71–80, 1999

Kinirons MT, Crome P: Clinical pharmacokinetic considerations in the elderly: an update. Clin Pharmacokinet 33:302–312, 1997

Kinzie JD, Leung P, Boehnlein J, et al: Tricyclic antidepressant plasma levels in Indochinese refugees: cultural and clinical implications. J Nerv Ment Dis 175:480–485, 1987

Kirsch I: Changing Expectations: A Key to Effective Psychotherapy. Pacific Grove, CA, Brooks/Cole, 1990

Kleinman A: Rethinking Psychiatry. New York, Free Press, 1988

Kleinman A, Eisenberg L, Good BJ: Culture, illness, and care: clinical lessons from anthropologic and cross-cultural research. Ann Intern Med 88:251–258, 1978

Landy D: Culture, Disease, and Healing. New York, Macmillan, 1977

Leads from the MMWR. Lead poisoning from Mexican folk remedies— California (letter). JAMA 250:3149, 1983

Leathart JB, London SJ, Steward A, et al: CYP2D6 phenotype-genotype relationships in African-Americans and Caucasians in Los Angeles. Pharmacogenetics 8:529–541, 1998

Lee S, Wing YK, Wong KC: Knowledge and compliance towards lithium therapy among Chinese psychiatric patients in Hong Kong. Aust N Z J Psychiatry 26:444–449, 1992

Leslie C: Asian Medical Systems: A Comparative Study. Berkeley, CA, University of California Press, 1976

Lewis W, Kennelly E, Bass G: Ritualistic use of the holly *Ilex guayusa* by Amazonian Jivaro Indians. J Ethnopharmacol 33:25–30, 1991

Li T, Vallada H, Curtis D, et al: Catechol-*O*-methyltransferase Val158Met polymorphism: frequency analysis in Han Chinese subjects and allelic association of the low activity allele with bipolar affective disorder. Pharmacogenetics 7:349–353, 1997

Lin K-M: Traditional Chinese medical beliefs and their relevance for mental illness and psychiatry, in Normal and Abnormal Behavior in Chinese Culture. Edited by Kleinman S, Lin TY. Boston, Reidel, 1981, pp 11–24

Lin K-M, Cheung F: Mental health issues for Asian-Americans. Psychiatr Serv 50:774–780, 1999

Lin K-M, Poland RE: Ethnicity, Culture, and Psychopharmacology, in Psychopharmacology: The Fourth Generation of Progress. Edited by Bloom FE, Kupfer DI. New York, Raven, 1995, pp 1907–1917

Lin K-M, DeMonteverde L, Nuccio I: Religion, healing and mental health among Filipino-Americans. International Journal of Mental Health 19:40–44, 1990

Lin K-M, Poland RE, Nakasaki G (eds): Psychopharmacology and Psychobiology of Ethnicity. Washington, DC, American Psychiatric Press, 1993

Lin K-M, Smith MW, Mendoza RP: Psychopharmacology in cross-cultural psychiatry, in Cross Cultural Psychiatry. Edited by Herrera JM, Lawson WB, Sramek JJ. New York, Wiley, 1999, pp 45–52

Littlewood R: Psychiatric diagnosis and racial bias: empirical and interpretative approaches. Soc Sci Med 34:141–149, 1992

Liu G: Effects of some compounds isolated from Chinese medicinal herbs on hepatic microsomal cytochrome P-450 and their potential biological consequences. Drug Metab Rev 23:439–465, 1991

Lopez SR: Patient variable biases in clinical judgment: conceptual overview and methodological considerations. Psychol Bull 106:184–203, 1989

Manji HK, Potter WZ, Lenox RH, et al: Signal transduction pathways: molecular targets for lithium's actions. Arch Gen Psychiatry 52:531–543, 1995

Manne SL, Jacobsen PB, Gorfinkle K, et al: Treatment adherence difficulties among children with cancer: the role of parenting style. J Pediatr Psychol 18(1):47–62, 1993

Marquez C, Taintor Z, Schwartz MA: Diagnosis of manic depressive illness in blacks. Compr Psychiatry 26:337–341, 1985

Marsella AJ, DeVos G, Hsu FLK: Culture and Self: Asian and Western Perspectives. New York, Tavistock, 1985

Marwick C: Scientists stress biodiversity–human health links. JAMA 273:1246, 1995

Masimirembwa CM, Hasler JA: Genetic polymorphism of drug metabolising enzymes in African populations: implications for the use of neuroleptics and antidepressants. Brain Res Bull 44:561–571, 1997

McLeod HL, Fang L, Luo X, et al: Ethnic differences in erythrocyte catechol-O-methyltransferase activity in black and white Americans. J Pharmacol Exp Ther 270:26–29, 1994

Mendoza R, Wan Y, Poland RE, et al: CYP2D6 polymorphism in a Mexican American population: relationship between genotyping and phenotyping. Submitted for publication

Mezzich JE, Kleinman A, Fabrega H, et al: Culture and Psychiatric Diagnosis. Washington, DC, American Psychiatric Press, 1995

Michaelovsky E, Frisch A, Rockah R, et al: A novel allele in the promoter region of the human serotonin transporter gene. Mol Psychiatry 4:97–99, 1999

Moerman D: Anthropology of symbolic healing. Currents in Anthropology 20:59–80, 1979

Morgenstern H, Glazer WM: Identifying risk factors for tardive dyskinesia among long-term outpatients maintained with neuroleptic medications. Arch Gen Psychiatry 50:723–733, 1993

Mukherjee S, Shukla S, Woodle J, et al: Misdiagnosis of schizophrenia in bipolar patients: a multiethnic comparison. Am J Psychiatry 140:1571–1574, 1983

National Institute of Mental Health: Genetics and Mental Disorders: Report of the National Institute of Mental Health's Genetics Workgroup. Available at: http://www.nimh.nih.gov/research/genetics.htm. Accessed July 14, 1999

Noble EP, Blum K, Ritchie T, et al: Allelic association of the D2 dopamine receptor gene with receptor-binding characteristics in alcoholism. Arch Gen Psychiatry 48:648–654, 1991

Oesterheld J, Kallepalli BR: Grapefruit juice and clomipramine: shifting metabolic ratios. J Clin Psychopharmacol 17:62–63, 1997

Okpaku SO: Clinical Methods in Transcultural Psychiatry. Washington, DC, American Psychiatric Press, 1998

Parsian A, Chakraverty S, Fisher L, et al: No association between polymorphisms in the human dopamine D3 and D4 receptors genes and alcoholism. Am J Med Genet 74:281–285, 1997

Pi EH, Gutierrez MA, Gray GE: Tardive dyskinesia: cross-cultural perspectives, in Psychopharmacology and Psychobiology of Ethnicity. Edited by Lin K-M, Poland RE, Nakasaki G. Washington, DC, American Psychiatric Press, 1993, pp 153–167

Polednak A: Racial and Ethnic Differences in Disease. New York, Oxford University Press, 1989

Price N, Glazer WM, Morgenstern H: Race and the use of fluphenazine decanoate. Am J Psychiatry 142:1491–1492, 1985

Rappaport H: The tenacity of folk psychotherapy: a functional interpretation. Social Psychiatry 12:127–132, 1977

Rivera-Calimlim L, Reilly DK: Difference in erythrocyte catechol-O-methyltransferase activity between Orientals and Caucasians: difference in levodopa tolerance. Clin Pharmacol Ther 35:804–809, 1984

Roh HK, Dahl ML, Johansson I, et al: Debrisoquine and S-mephenytoin hydroxylation phenotypes and genotypes in a Korean population. Pharmacogenetics 6:441–447, 1996

Ross P, Hall L, Smirnov I, et al: High level multiplex genotyping by MALDI-TOF mass spectrometry. Nat Biotechnol 16:1347–1351, 1998

Roukema R, Fadem BH, James B, et al: Bipolar disorder in a low socioeconomic population: difficulties in diagnosis. J Nerv Ment Dis 72:76–79, 1984

Sackett D, Haynes R: Compliance With Therapeutic Regimens. Baltimore, MD, Johns Hopkins University Press, 1976

Salzman C: Clinical Geriatric Psychopharmacology. New York, McGraw-Hill, 1984

Sander T, Harms H, Podschus J, et al: Dopamine D1, D2 and D3 receptor genes in alcohol dependence. Psychiatr Genet 5:171–176, 1995

Shepherd M: The placebo: from specificity to the non-specific and back. Psychol Med 23:569–578, 1993

Smeraldi E, Zanardi R, Benedetti F, et al: Polymorphism within the promoter of the serotonin transporter gene and antidepressant efficacy of fluvoxamine. Mol Psychiatry 3:508–511, 1998

Smith M, Lin K-M, Mendoza R: Nonbiological issues affecting psychopharmacotherapy: cultural considerations, in Psychopharmacology and Psychobiology of Ethnicity. Edited by Lin K-M, Poland RE, Nakasaki G. Washington, DC, American Psychiatric Press, 1993, pp 37–58

Sramek J, Roy S, Ahrens T, et al: Prevalence of tardive dyskinesia among three ethnic groups of chronic psychiatric patients. Hospital and Community Psychiatry 42:590–592, 1991

Stephens EA, Taylor JA, Yang CH, et al: Ethnic variation in the CYP2E1 gene: polymorphism analysis of 695 African-Americans, European-Americans and Taiwanese. Pharmacogenetics 4:185–192, 1994

Strickland TL, Ranganath V, Lin KM, et al: Psychopharmacologic considerations in the treatment of black American populations. Psychopharmacol Bull 27:441–448, 1991

Sue S, Fujino DC, Hu LT, et al: Community mental health services for ethnic minority groups: a test of the cultural responsiveness hypothesis. J Consult Clin Psychol 59:533–540, 1991

Sullivan PF, Fifield WJ, Kennedy MA, et al: No association between novelty seeking and the type 4 dopamine receptor gene *(DRD4)* in two New Zealand samples. Am J Psychiatry 155:98–101, 1998

Swartz R, Burgoyne K, Smith M, et al: Tardive dyskinesia and ethnicity: review of the literature. Ann Clin Psychiatry 9:53–59, 1997

Swartzman LC, Burkell J: Expectations and the placebo effect in clinical drug trials: why we should not turn a blind eye to unblinding, and other cautionary notes. Clin Pharmacol Ther 64:1–7, 1998

Tanaka E: In vivo age-related changes in hepatic drug-oxidizing capacity in humans. J Clin Pharm Ther 23:247–255, 1998

Tinsley H, Bowman S, Ray S: Manipulation of expectancies about counseling and psychotherapy: review and analysis of expectancy manipulation strategies and results. Journal of Counseling Psychology 35:99–108, 1988

Vandenbergh DJ, Persico AM, Hawkins AL, et al: Human dopamine transporter gene (DAT1) maps to chromosome 5p15.3 and displays a VNTR. Genomics 14:1104–1106, 1992

Vermeer DE, Ferrell RE Jr: Nigerian geophagical clay: a traditional antidiarrheal pharmaceutical. Science 227:634–636, 1985

Wang SL, Huang JD, Lai MD, et al: Molecular basis of genetic variation in debrisoquin hydroxylation in Chinese subjects: polymorphism in RFLP and DNA sequence of CYP2D6. Clin Pharmacol Ther 53:410–418, 1993

Weber WW: Pharmacogenetics. New York, Oxford University Press, 1997

Weiner M, Weiner GJ: The kinetics and dynamics of responses to placebo. Clin Pharmacol Ther 60:247–254, 1996

Weiss M: Explanatory Model Interview Catalogue (EMIC): framework for comparative study of illness. Transcultural Psychiatry 34:235–263, 1997

Westermeyer J: Psychiatric Care of Migrants: A Clinical Guide. Washington, DC, American Psychiatric Press, 1989

Wetzel MS, Eisenberg DM, Kaptchuk TJ: Courses involving complementary and alternative medicine at US medical schools. JAMA 280:784–787, 1998

White L, Tursky B, Schwartz GE: Placebo: Theory, Research, and Mechanisms. New York, Guilford, 1985

Wig NN: Indian concepts of mental health and their impact on care of the mentally ill. International Journal of Mental Health 18:71–80, 1989

Wolffers I: Traditional practitioners' behavioral adaptations to changing patients' demands in Sri Lanka. Soc Sci Med 29:1111–1119, 1989

Yamahara J, Kobayashi M, Matsuda H: Anticholinergic action of *Swertia japonica* and an active constituent. J Ethnopharmacol 33:31–35, 1991

Chapter 2

Issues in Pharmacotherapy for African Americans

William B. Lawson, M.D., Ph.D., F.A.P.A.

African Americans generally have limited access to the mental health system or receive suboptimal treatment (Flaherty and Meagher 1980; Lawson et al. 1994). Pharmacotherapy is among these suboptimal treatments. Multiple studies have shown that for the most part, African Americans are either undertreated or treated inappropriately (Lawson 1996; Strickland et al. 1991). They are more likely to receive antipsychotic medication, and higher doses of medication across diagnostic categories, leading to more adverse consequences (Chung et al. 1995; Lawson 1986a; Segal et al. 1996; Strakowski et al. 1993). In this chapter, I show that socio-economic, cultural, attitudinal, and biological factors interact to prevent optimal care for African Americans.

Affective Disorders

An extensive literature shows that African Americans with affective disorders are often undertreated or treated inappropriately with antipsychotic medications (Lawson 1996; Strickland et al. 1991). A contributory factor is the underdiagnosis of affective disorders. Diagnoses of schizophrenia instead of affective disorders are often made in African Americans (Adebimpe 1994), despite widespread use of DSM-IV (American Psychiatric Association 1994) and evidence from epidemiological studies. Using reliable and established diagnostic interview methods, large multisite studies have consistently found that ethnic differences in prevalence of mental disorders are modest at best (Kessler et al. 1994; Robins et al. 1991). Nevertheless, many clinicians believe that affective disorders are uncommon in African Americans (Jones and Gray 1986).

Bipolar affective disorder is often misdiagnosed in African Americans, leading to a delay in the initiation of appropriate anti-manic treatment. Studies more than a decade ago found that African Americans with clear evidence of bipolar disorder were more likely to receive a diagnosis of schizophrenia and were less likely to undergo lithium therapy than Caucasians (Bell and Mehta 1980, 1981; Mukherjee et al. 1983). More recent studies have shown that manic subtypes such as mixed mania, rapid-cycling mania, and mania with psychotic features may be more common than pure mania (Bowden 1995). These subtypes may be more lithium resistant. The earlier studies involved patients with uncomplicated bipolar I disorder. Given the literature, one could presume that these other subtypes may be more commonly misdiagnosed in African Americans. Unfortunately, there are no reports of recent studies examining ethnic differences in bipolar subtypes or treatment response of those subtypes.

Depressive disorders may also be misdiagnosed. African Americans with psychotic depression are more likely than Caucasians to have their condition diagnosed as schizophrenia (Raskin et al. 1975). We reported that Hispanics with psychotic depression are at increased risk of receiving a diagnosis of schizophrenia (Lawson 1990; Lawson et al. 1992). We studied a group of Mexican American patients for whom English was a second language and in whom the presumptive diagnosis was schizophrenia. Using a Spanish translator, we found that half of the patients met DSM-III-R (American Psychiatric Association 1987) criteria for delusional depression. These patients had been treated exclusively with antipsychotics. When an antidepressant was added to their treatment, they improved and were able to be discharged.

Often, however, the diagnosis of major depression is not made. Several large studies have shown that African Americans with major depression receive a diagnosis only 50% of the time (Brown et al. 1995; Sussman et al. 1987). Probably a much smaller percentage are adequately treated.

Unwillingness to seek treatment in the mental health system is another reason African Americans receive suboptimal therapy. African Americans who are in distress or depressed often do not seek professional help (Brown et al. 1995; Neighbors 1984; Sussman et al. 1987). When treatment is sought, it is usually sought after a delay. Treatment often is sought not from mental health professionals but from primary care providers, family members, friends, or the faith community. With the exception of the primary care providers, help is sought from individuals unfamiliar with the pharmacotherapy of depression.

Fear of hospitalization and involuntary commitment is often the reason given for avoiding treatment (Sussman et al. 1987). Unfortunately, there is some truth in that belief. African Americans are more likely to be hospitalized or involuntarily committed (Flaherty and Meagher 1980; Lawson et al. 1994; Lindsey et al. 1989; Paul and Menditto 1992; Strakowski et al. 1995). Consequently, African Americans have a different perception of the mental health system, often not seeing it as a resource for consensual treatment.

The prevalence of mental disorders among African Americans may be similar to that among other groups, but African Americans may present with different symptoms, symptoms that would contribute to the misdiagnosis of schizophrenia and increased likelihood of antipsychotic use. A consistent finding is the greater likelihood of psychotic symptoms in African Americans for a range of affective and anxiety disorders. African Americans with bipolar disorder are more likely to have psychotic symptoms such as hallucinations (Strakowski et al. 1996), and those experiencing mania may present with more irritable symptoms, which could be misinterpreted as psychosis. In African Americans with depression, the existence of more paranoid symptoms may be indicated by the Minnesota Multiphasic Personality Inventory (MMPI) (Adebimpe et al. 1979). Suspiciousness is seen more often than in Caucasians and is interpreted by some as a "healthy paranoia" (Jones and Gray 1986). Consequently, antipsychotics may be used more frequently in African Americans because they are seen as being in need of treatment for psychotic symptoms.

Anxiety Disorders

Recent studies have shown that African Americans with various anxiety disorders are also likely to be given a misdiagnosis of psychosis and are more likely to receive antipsychotic treatment. Panic disorder and phobic disorders are often underdiagnosed in African Americans, despite some evidence that these disorders may be more common in ethnic minorities (Brown et al. 1990; Neal and Turner 1991; Paradis et al. 1994). The individual undergoing a panic attack could be perceived as having hallucinatory or delusional fears and could receive a diagnosis of psychosis rather than of an anxiety disorder (Lawson 1999).

Obsessive-compulsive disorder is rarely diagnosed in African Americans (Friedman et al. 1993; Hatch et al. 1992; Paradis et al. 1994). Although there are no definitive studies, case reports suggest that many of these patients are diagnosed as being psychotic (Lawson 1999). The ego-dystonic obsessions in obsessive-compulsive disorder may easily be misinterpreted as delusions or a thought disturbance, and the compulsions may be mistaken for psychotic behavior (Hwang and Hollander 1993).

Recent studies have shown that posttraumatic stress disorder (PTSD) in African Americans may be associated with different symptoms and may be misdiagnosed, with the consequent greater likelihood of antipsychotic treatment (Lawson 1999). In all populations, typical symptoms in PTSD may easily be mistaken for psychotic symptoms. Flashbacks in patients with PTSD may be mistaken for hallucinatory experiences, emotional blunting for a flattened affect, and hyperreactivity for psychotic excitement. Consequently, patients are at risk of being misdiagnosed with schizophrenia (Allen 1996).

Symptom presentation may differ in African Americans with combat-related PTSD compared with Caucasians and Hispanics with the disorder (Allen 1996; Penk and Allen 1991). African American substance abusers with heavy-combat exposure were reported to be more disturbed than a similar group of whites and scored higher on the MMPI scales for paranoid and psychotic symptoms (Penk et al. 1989). A later study found higher levels of psychotic symptoms and paranoid ideation among blacks with PTSD compared with whites with the disorder, using the MMPI-2 groups (Frueh et al. 1996). Unlike the older MMPI, the MMPI-2 (Hathaway and McKinley 1989) was normed on diverse ethnic groups.

Consistent with these findings, African American veterans reportedly received more neuroleptic medication than did Hispanics or whites, either while hospitalized or at the time of discharge (White and Faustman 1989). Together these findings suggest that the different presentation by African Americans with PTSD, who perhaps present with more psychotic symptoms, might contribute to the overdiagnosing of schizophrenia and could contribute to an increased likelihood of antipsychotic treatment.

Schizophrenia

African Americans with schizophrenia or other severe mental disorders are often treated differently in the mental health system. As noted earlier, they are more likely to be hospitalized, involuntarily committed, or placed in seclusion or restraints (Flaherty and Meagher 1980; Lawson et al. 1994; Lindsey et al. 1989; Paul and Menditto 1992; Soloff and Turner 1982; Strakowski et al. 1995). Moreover, African Americans are more likely than Caucasians to receive medication and higher doses of antipsychotic medication, per nurse request (Chung et al. 1995; Flaherty and Meagher 1980; Lawson 1986a; Strakowski et al. 1993). A common factor may be the tendency of African Americans to delay in obtaining treatment or to seek mental health treatment only as a last resort. African Americans have a different experience in the mental health system, which may have an impact on treatment acceptability. They are more likely to receive depot medication, which suggests a history of noncompliance and lack of investment in mental health treatment (Price et al. 1985; Segal et al. 1996).

Therapist attitudes may directly affect care. African Americans' treatments are terminated sooner by Caucasian therapists, especially if the therapist is racially biased (Chung et al. 1995; Flaherty and Meagher 1980; Yamamoto et al. 1967). Conversely, African American patients with African American providers stay in treatment longer (Rosenheck et al. 1995). African Americans are also more likely to be perceived as being violent or dangerous. We reported that the staff on an inpatient unit perceived African American patients to be more dangerous even though independent assessment of violent behavior showed that these patients were significantly less likely to be violent toward themselves or others (Lawson et al. 1984). Segal et al. (1996) attempted to determine whether therapists' feelings about their schizophrenic patients affected prescribing of medication for them. The investigators reported that African Americans received more psychiatric medication, more doses of antipsychotic medications, more injections of antipsychotic medication, and higher 24-hour doses than did whites. Prescribing patterns were related to the willingness of the physician to engage patients in treatment. Unwillingness to engage was associated with excessive medicating. Presumably, social distance (most of the providers were white) increased the likelihood that patients would receive more medication. Taken together, these findings suggest that therapists' attitudes and perceptions of their patients' racial identities can affect treatment.

Pharmacological Factors and Adverse Events

Examination of pharmacokinetic and pharmacodynamic factors can help to determine whether ethnic differences in dosing have a biological basis. Previous studies showed that Asian providers often prescribed lower doses of many different psychotropic agents, including antipsychotic medications and tricyclic antidepressants (TCAs), to Asian patients (Lin and Finder 1983; Yamashita and Asano 1979). Part of the reason for this prescribing of lower doses is that Asians report more side effects and have higher plasma levels than do Caucasians given the same oral doses (Bond 1991; Lin et al. 1993). A review of the literature suggests that African Americans also show differences in medication response, but these differences do not appear to affect dosing patterns.

Antidepressants

Early multicenter studies showed that African Americans tend to respond more quickly to antipsychotic medication and TCAs than do Caucasian patients (Lawson 1986a). Other studies have found an increased risk of toxic side effects and higher plasma levels of TCAs in African Americans than in whites (Ziegler and Biggs 1977). Rudorfer and Robins (1982) showed that African Americans who had taken lethal doses of TCAs had higher plasma levels than did whites who had overdosed. These findings suggest that

African Americans may be at a greater risk for toxic side effects when treated with TCAs (Silver et al. 1993).

These differences in clinical response and pharmacokinetics have been attributed to ethnic differences in drug metabolism mediated through the cytochrome P450 microsomal enzyme system, which is responsible for the metabolism of most of the older psychotropic medications, including typical antipsychotics and TCAs (Lin et al. 1993; Silver et al. 1993). Earlier studies showed that Caucasians were more likely than Asians and African Americans to be poor metabolizers of psychotropic medication, a finding inconsistent with clinical experience, because poor metabolizers should require less medication. However, new mutations have recently been discovered in the enzymatic systems of the latter groups that are intermediate in the rate of metabolism. Thus, up to 47%–70% of African Americans and Asian Americans may be slow metabolizers, which could account for the higher incidence of side effects (Mendoza et al. 1999).

New pharmacotherapeutic approaches may prevent some of the consequences of prescribing excessive doses of psychotropic medication. As noted earlier, African Americans with depression may have more side effects and develop toxicity more easily when treated with TCAs. Moreover, TCAs present a special problem for all ethnic groups because these agents are cardiotoxic. Consequently, the clinician is often in the dilemma of giving a toxic agent to a person at risk for suicide. Newer agents such as serotonin reuptake inhibitors (SSRIs) do not have the side-effect profile of older agents and, in particular, they are associated with almost no cardiovascular toxicity (Frazer 1997; Preskorn 1995). Consequently, SSRIs are far safer, which is especially important given the risk of toxicity of TCAs among ethnic minorities. Many of the newer SSRIs have less effect on the hepatic P450 system, which might further reduce the likelihood of overdose and toxicity for ethnic minorities (Preskorn 1995, 1997).

Antimanics

Relatively recent studies suggest that African Americans handle lithium differently than do other ethnic groups. A higher red blood cell–to-plasma ratio of lithium has been consistently found in African Americans (Okpaku et al. 1980; Strickland et al. 1993, 1995). The clinical significance was unknown until recently. Strickland et al. (1995) found that African Americans taking lithium reported more side effects during a standardized interview than did whites. Moreover, side-effect ratings were directly related to red blood cell–to-plasma ratio. Dr. Keh-Min Lin's group (K.-M. Lin, personal communication, May 1999) recently replicated this finding. Other reports suggest an increased risk of other side effects with a high plasma-to–red blood cell ratio such as lithium neuroleptic toxicity (Strickland et al. 1993). It is not clear whether African Americans require lower clinical doses, but caution is certainly warranted.

These findings have important implications for the treatment of bipolar affective disorder. Some agents used to treat partial-complex seizures such as carbamazepine and various valproate formulations have been found to be effective in bipolar affective disorder (Bowden 1995). One such agent, divalproex, is now the most commonly prescribed antimanic agent. These agents may be more effective in subtypes of mania that are not lithium responsive. As noted earlier, African Americans are more often prescribed antipsychotics. Poor tolerance of lithium may be a factor. Improving access to alternatives to lithium may reduce the need for antipsychotics in some African Americans with mania.

Antipsychotics

Tardive dyskinesia (TD) remains a major side effect of antipsychotic medication. Ethnicity is one of several factors that determine the likelihood of development of TD. Glazer and colleagues (Glazer et al. 1994; Morgenstern and Glazer 1993) reported that African American patients were more likely to develop TD than were Caucasian patients. One possibility is that African Americans may have an unrecognized genetic or enzymatic defect that may predispose them to TD (e.g., a defect that results in higher plasma levels of the antipsychotic agent). African Americans are, however, more likely to receive pharmacotherapy differently.

As indicated earlier, African Americans are more likely than whites to receive neuroleptic medication in general and to receive higher neuroleptic doses. Dosing is more likely to be intermittent because of orders to take the medication as needed, frequent medication interruptions due to poor compliance, or lack of access to regular treatment. Exposure to neuroleptic medication, excessive dosing, and intermittent treatment are all risk factors for TD (Kane et al. 1992). Finally, in neuroleptic-exposed individuals, a diagnosis of an affective disorder is another risk factor for TD. As noted previously, African Americans with affective disorders are at greater risk of receiving antipsychotic medication. In a study involving elderly schizophrenic patients (Lindamer et al. 1999), the rate of TD was 47% among African Americans and 26% among whites. Neuroleptic exposure was well controlled, which suggests that there may be an unknown biological risk factor.

Newer antipsychotic agents may also be helpful with regard to these concerns. The atypical antipsychotic clozapine was the first of the atypical antipsychotics, which offer significant advantages over typical antipsychotics (Kane et al. 1988). Clozapine is effective in many patients unresponsive to treatment with typical antipsychotics. It also seems to be associated with few extrapyramidal symptoms (EPS) and a lower risk for TD. However, other features of the drug limit its use by African Americans.

Clozapine therapy is expensive (Griffith 1990). Part of the high cost is due to the significantly greater risk of agranulocytosis associated with treatment, which has led to the requirement of regular blood monitoring (Alvir et al. 1993). It is recommended that patients have minimum leukocyte counts before clozapine therapy is initiated, despite the lack of evidence that preexisting white blood cell counts predict development of agranulocytosis. However, in African Americans, normal leukocyte counts may be well below listed normal values ("benign leukopenia") (Caramihai et al. 1975; Karayalcin et al. 1972). As a result, the overly cautious clinician may choose not to prescribe clozapine to otherwise healthy African American patients. Moeller and associates (1995) reported that African Americans are less likely to receive clozapine.

Other new atypical antipsychotics are not associated with an increased risk of agranulocytosis (unlike typical antipsychotics), are less likely to cause acute EPS, and probably are associated with a lesser risk of TD. Risperidone, another atypical agent, is not associated with an excessive risk of agranulocytosis but is highly effective, with a low incidence of EPS (Marder and Meibach 1994). Hispanic patients given risperidone responded more rapidly than did non-Hispanic patients who received the same drug (Frackiewicz et al. 1999). Although they experienced more EPS than non-Hispanics did, Hispanic patients treated with risperidone had fewer such side effects than those treated with typical antipsychotics.

Another atypical agent, olanzapine, also is associated with lower rates of EPS and TD and is not associated with a high risk for agranulocytosis (Tollefson et al. 1997). In a multisite study, EPS and dyskinesia occurred in a smaller percentage of patients of African descent who took olanzapine (4%) than in similar patients who took haloperidol (22%) (Tran et al. 1999). In addition, significant ethnic differences in movement-disordered events were seen with haloperidol therapy but not with olanzapine therapy.

Research and Accessibility

Additional research is needed to develop novel agents that are better tolerated by African Americans and other ethnic minorities. Older agents often have unacceptable side effects. Newer agents demonstrate that ethnic minorities do not need to experience unacceptable side effects. Unfortunately, African Americans are often underrepresented in clinical trials involving newer agents or as investigators (Lawson 1986a; Svensson 1989). A contributing factor to an unwillingness by African Americans to become involved in mental health research is widespread awareness of the Tuskegee study (Roy 1995). In this federally sponsored study, which was begun in the 1930s, African American men with a diagnosis of syphilis had treatment withheld without their knowledge. Only newspaper exposés in the 1970s ended the study. As a consequence, psychotropic medication and mental health treatment are often viewed with suspicion by African Americans.

New treatments often are more costly than treatments with standard agents, because pharmaceutical manufacturers try to recoup development costs for drugs that are patent protected. Costs are a significant barrier for African Americans. Twenty-two percent of African Americans live below the federal poverty line, the median income of African Americans is 60% that of Caucasians, and, most important, the net worth of African Americans is only one-tenth that of whites, reflecting the fact that most African Americans are only one or two generations from poverty (Lawson 1986b; O'Hare et al. 1991). As a result, African Americans are more likely to be uninsured, depend on public facilities for care, or depend on public insurance programs such as state disability programs or Medicaid (Snowden and Cheung 1990). Medicaid and public facilities tend to have restrictions that can limit the availability of new agents because of cost, despite newer evidence that psychotropic agents are often cost effective (Rosenheck et al. 1997). Because of costs, newer agents are often used as second-line therapy. Yet the findings previously described provide compelling evidence for making many of these agents more accessible to African Americans.

Conclusion

African Americans receive differential, often substandard treatment in many mental health systems. Many of these concerns could be addressed with new advances in diagnosis and treatment. More must be done to educate providers about the need to address cultural issues and to provide optimal care to all patients. More needs to be done in treatment management to avoid two tiers of care as controlling costs continues to be a high priority. Finally, African Americans should have equal access to services and should benefit equally from advances that have occurred in mental health care.

References

Adebimpe VR: Race, racism, and epidemiological surveys. Hospital and Community Psychiatry 45:27–31, 1994

Allen IM: PTSD among African Americans, in Ethnocultural Aspects of Posttraumatic Stress Disorder: Issues, Research, and Clinical Applications. Edited by Marsella AJ, Friedman MJ, Gerrity ET, et al. Washington, DC, American Psychological Association, 1996, pp 209–238

Alvir JMJ, Lieberman JA, Safferman AZ, et al: Clozapine-induced agranulocytosis: incidence and risk factors in the United States. N Engl J Med 329:162–167, 1993

American Psychiatric Association: Diagnostic and Statistical Manual of Mental Disorders, 3rd Edition, Revised. Washington, DC, American Psychiatric Association, 1987

American Psychiatric Association: Diagnostic and Statistical Manual of Mental Disorders, 4th Edition. Washington, DC, American Psychiatric Association, 1994

Bell CC, Mehta H: The misdiagnosis of black patients with manic depressive illness. J Natl Med Assoc 72:141–145, 1980

Bell CC, Mehta H: Misdiagnosis of black patients with manic depressive illness: second in a series. J Natl Med Assoc 73:101–107, 1981

Bond WS: Ethnicity and psychotropic drugs. Clin Pharm 10:467–470, 1991

Bowden CL: Predictors of response to divalproex and lithium. J Clin Psychiatry 56 (suppl 3):25–30, 1995

Brown DR, Eaton WW, Sussman L: Racial differences in prevalence of phobic disorders. J Nerv Ment Dis 178:434–441, 1990

Brown DR, Feroz A, Gary LE, et al: Major depression in a community of African Americans. Am J Psychiatry 152:373–378, 1995

Caramihai E, Karayalcin G, Aballi AJ, et al: Leukocyte count differences in healthy white and black children 1 to 5 years of age. J Pediatr 86:252–254, 1975

Chung H, Mahler JC, Kakuna T: Racial differences in the treatment of psychiatric inpatients. Psychiatr Serv 46:586–591, 1995

Flaherty JA, Meagher R: Measuring racial bias in inpatient treatment. Am J Psychiatry 137:679–682, 1980

Frackiewicz E, Sramek JJ, Collazo Y, et al: Risperidone in the treatment of Hispanic schizophrenic patients, in Cross Cultural Psychiatry. Edited by Herrera JM, Lawson WB, Sramek JJ. New York, Wiley, 1999, pp 183–192

Frazer A: Pharmacology of antidepressants. J Clin Psychopharmacol 17(suppl 1):2S–18S, 1997

Friedman S, Hatch ML, Paradis C, et al: Obsessive-compulsive disorder in two black ethnic groups: incidence in an urban dermatology clinic. J Anxiety Disord 7:343–348, 1993

Frueh BC, Smith DW, Libet JM: Racial differences on psychological measures in combat veterans seeking treatment for PTSD. J Pers Assess 66:41–53, 1996

Glazer WM, Morgenstern H, Doucette J: Race and tardive dyskinesia among outpatients at a CMHC. Hospital and Community Psychiatry 45:38–42, 1994

Griffith EEH: Clozapine: problems for the public sector (editorial). Hospital and Community Psychiatry 41:837, 1990

Hatch ML, Paradis C, Friedman S, et al: Obsessive-compulsive disorder in patients with chronic pruritic conditions: case studies and discussion. J Am Acad Dermatol 26:549–551, 1992

Hathaway SR, McKinley JC: Minnesota Multiphasic Personality Inventory—2. Minneapolis, MN, University of Minnesota, 1989

Hwang MY, Hollander E: Schizo-obsessive disorders. Psychiatric Annals 23:396–401, 1993

Jones BE, Gray BA: Problems in diagnosing schizophrenia and affective disorders among blacks. Hospital and Community Psychiatry 37:61–65, 1986

Kane J, Honigfeld G, Singer J, et al: Clozapine for the treatment-resistant schizophrenic: a double-blind comparison with chlorpromazine. Arch Gen Psychiatry 45:789–796, 1988

Kane JM, Jeste DV, Barnes TRE, et al: Tardive Dyskinesia: A Task Force Report of the American Psychiatric Association. Washington, DC, American Psychiatric Association, 1992

Karayalcin G, Rosner F, Sawitsky A: Pseudoneutropenia in Negroes: a normal phenomenon. N Y State J Med 72:1815–1817, 1972

Kessler RC, McGonagle KA, Zhao S, et al: Lifetime and 12-month prevalence of DSM-III-R psychiatric disorders in the United States. Results from the National Comorbidity Survey. Arch Gen Psychiatry 51:8–19, 1994

Lawson WB: Racial and ethnic factors in psychiatric research. Hospital and Community Psychiatry 37:50–54, 1986a

Lawson WB: The black family and chronic mental illness. American Journal of Social Psychiatry 6:57–61, 1986b

Lawson WB: Clinical issues in the pharmacotherapy of African-Americans. Psychopharmacol Bull 32:275–281, 1996

Lawson WB: Psychiatric diagnosis of African Americans, in Cross Cultural Psychiatry. Edited by Herrera JM, Lawson WB, Sramek JJ. New York, Wiley, 1999, pp 99–104

Lawson WB, Yesavage JA, Werner RD: Race, violence, and psychopathology. J Clin Psychiatry 45:294–297, 1984

Lawson WB, Herrera JM, Costa J: The dexamethasone suppression test as an adjunct in diagnosing depression. J Assoc Acad Minor Phys 3:17–19, 1992

Lawson WB, Hepler N, Holladay J, et al: Race as a factor in inpatient and outpatient admissions and diagnosis. Hospital and Community Psychiatry 45:72–74, 1994

Lin K-M, Finder E: Neuroleptic dosage for Asians. Am J Psychiatry 140:490–491, 1983

Lin K-M, Poland RE, Silver B: Overview: the interface between psychobiology and ethnicity, in Psychopharmacology and Psychobiology of Ethnicity. Edited by Lin K-M, Poland RE, Nakasaki G. Washington, DC, American Psychiatric Press, 1993, pp 11–35

Lindamer L, Lacro JP, Jeste DV: Relationship of ethnicity to the effects of antipsychotic medication, in Cross Cultural Psychiatry. Edited by Herrera JM, Lawson WB, Sramek JJ. New York, Wiley, 1999, pp 193–203

Lindsey KP, Paul GL, Mariotto MJ: Urban psychiatric commitments: disability and dangerous behavior of black and white recent admissions. Hospital and Community Psychiatry 40:286–294, 1989

Marder SR, Meibach RC: Risperidone in the treatment of schizophrenia. Am J Psychiatry 151:825–835, 1994

Mendoza RP, Smith MW, Lin K-M: Ethnicity and the pharmacogenetics of drug-metabolizing enzymes, in Cross Cultural Psychiatry. Edited by Herrera JM, Lawson WB, Sramek JJ. New York, Wiley, 1999, pp 3–15

Moeller FG, Chen YW, Steinberg JL, et al: Risk factors for clozapine discontinuation among 805 patients in the VA hospital system. Ann Clin Psychiatry 7:167–173, 1995

Morgenstern H, Glazer WM: Identifying risk factors for tardive dyskinesia among chronic outpatients maintained on neuroleptic medications: results of the Yale tardive dyskinesia study. Arch Gen Psychiatry 50:723–733, 1993

Mukherjee S, Shukla S, Woodline J: Misdiagnosis of schizophrenia in bipolar patients: a multi-ethnic comparison. Am J Psychiatry 140:1571–1574, 1983

Neal AM, Turner SM: Anxiety disorders research with African Americans: current status. Psychol Bull 109:400–410, 1991

Neighbors HW: The distribution of psychiatric morbidity in black Americans: a review and suggestion for research. Community Ment Health J 20:169–181, 1984

O'Hare WP, Pollard KM, Mann TL, et al: African Americans in the 1990's. Population Bulletin 46:1–40, 1991

Okpaku S, Frazer A, Mendels J: A pilot study of racial differences in erythrocyte lithium transport. Am J Psychiatry 137:120–121, 1980

Paradis CM, Hatch M, Friedman S: Anxiety disorders in African Americans: an update. J Natl Med Assoc 86:609–612, 1994

Parson ER: Ethnicity and traumatic stress: the intersecting point in psychotherapy, in Trauma and Its Wake: The Study and Treatment of Posttraumatic Stress Disorder. Edited by Figley CR. New York, Brunner/Mazel, 1985

Paul GI, Menditto AA: Effectiveness of inpatient treatment programs for mentally ill adults in public psychiatric facilities. Applied Preventive Psychology 1:41–63, 1992

Penk WE, Allen IM: Clinical assessment of post-traumatic stress disorder (PTSD) among American minorities who served in Vietnam. J Trauma Stress 4:41–66, 1991

Penk WE, Robinowitz R, Black J, et al: Ethnicity: post-traumatic stress disorder (PTSD) differences among black, white, and Hispanic veterans who differ in degrees of exposure to combat in Vietnam. J Clin Psychol 45:729–735, 1989

Preskorn SH: Comparison of the tolerability of bupropion, fluoxetine, imipramine, nefazodone, paroxetine, sertraline, and venlafaxine. J Clin Psychiatry 56(suppl 6):12–21, 1995

Preskorn SH: Selection of an antidepressant: mirtazapine. J Clin Psychiatry 58(suppl 6):3–8, 1997

Price N, Glazer W, Morgenstern H: Demographic predictors of the use of injectable versus oral antipsychotic medications in outpatients. Am J Psychiatry 142:1491–1492, 1985

Raskin A, Crook TH, Herman KD: Psychiatric history and symptom differences in black and white depressed inpatients. J Consult Clin Psychol 43:73–80, 1975

Robins LN, Locke B, Regier DA: An overview of psychiatric disorders in America, in Psychiatric Disorders in America: The Epidemologic Catchment Area Study. Edited by Robins LN, Regier DA. New York, Free Press, 1991, pp 328–366

Rosenheck R, Fontana A, Cottrol C: Effect of clinician-veteran racial pairing in the treatment of post traumatic stress disorder. Am J Psychiatry 152:555–563, 1995

Rosenheck R, Cramer J, Xu W, et al: A comparison of clozapine and haloperidol in hospitalized patients with refractory schizophrenia. N Engl J Med 337:809–815, 1997

Roy B: The Tuskegee syphilis experiment: biotechnology and the administrative state. J Natl Med Assoc 87:56–67, 1995

Rudorfer MV, Robins E: Amitriptyline overdose: clinical effects on tricyclic antidepressant plasma levels. J Clin Psychiatry 43:457–460, 1982

Segal SP, Bola J, Watson M: Race, quality of care, and antipsychotic prescribing practices in psychiatric emergency services. Psychiatr Serv 47:282–286, 1996

Silver B, Poland RE, Lin K-M: Ethnicity and the pharmacology of tricyclic antidepressants, in Psychopharmacology and Psychobiology of Ethnicity. Edited by Lin K-M, Poland RE, Nakasaki G. Washington, DC, American Psychiatric Press, 1993, pp 61–89

Snowden LR, Cheung FK: Use of inpatient mental health services by members of ethnic minority groups. Am Psychol 45:347–355, 1990

Soloff PA, Turner SM: Patterns of seclusion: a prospective study. J Nerv Ment Dis 169:37–44, 1982

Strakowski SM, Shelton RC, Kolbrener ML: The effects of race and co-morbidity on clinical diagnosis in patients with psychosis. J Clin Psychiatry 54:96–102, 1993

Strakowski SM, Lonczak HS, Sax K, et al: The effects of race on diagnosis and disposition from a psychiatric emergency service. J Clin Psychiatry 56:101–107, 1995

Strakowski SM, McElroy SL, Keck PE Jr, et al: Racial influence on diagnosis in psychotic mania. J Affect Disord 39:157–162, 1996

Strickland TL, Ranganath V, Lin K-M, et al: Psychopharmacologic considerations in the treatment of black American populations. Psychopharmacol Bull 27:441–448, 1991

Strickland TL, Lawson WB, Lin K-M: Interethnic variation in response to lithium therapy among African-American and Asian-American populations, in Psychopharmacology and Psychobiology of Ethnicity. Edited by Lin K-M, Poland RE, Nakasaki G. Washington, DC, American Psychiatric Press, 1993, pp 107–123

Strickland TL, Lin K-M, Fu P, et al: Comparison of lithium ratio between African-American and Caucasian bipolar patients. Biol Psychiatry 37:325–330, 1995

Sussman LK, Robins LN, Earls F: Treatment-seeking for depression by black and white Americans. Soc Sci Med 24:187–196, 1987

Svensson CK: Representation of American blacks in clinical trials of new drugs. JAMA 261:263–265, 1989

Tollefson GD, Beasley CM, Tran VP, et al: Olanzapine versus haloperidol in the treatment of schizophrenia and schizoaffective and schizophreniform disorders: results of an international collaborative trial. Am J Psychiatry 154:457–465, 1997

Tran PV, Lawson WB, Andersen S, et al: Treatment of the African American patient with novel antipsychotic agents, in Cross Cultural Psychiatry. Edited by Herrera JM, Lawson WB, Sramek JJ. New York, Wiley, 1999, pp 131–138

White PA, Faustman WO: PTSD in minorities. Hospital and Community Psychiatry 40:86–87, 1989

Yamamoto J, James QC, Bloombaum M, et al: Racial factors in patient selection. Am J Psychiatry 124:630–636, 1967

Yamashita I, Asano Y: Tricyclic antidepressants: therapeutic plasma level. Psychopharmacol Bull 15:40–41, 1979

Ziegler VE, Biggs JT: Tricyclic plasma levels: effect of age, race, sex and smoking. JAMA 238:2167–2169, 1977

Chapter 3

The Hispanic Response to Psychotropic Medications

Ricardo Mendoza, M.D.
Michael W. Smith, M.D.

Despite the growing importance of the Hispanic population, few studies of pharmacological response in this ethnic group have been conducted. Further, when the data available are analyzed, a common methodological problem is found. Hispanic subgroups have been lumped together in national and international clinical efficacy trials, and the data have subsequently been used in attempts to characterize a particular "Hispanic" response. Technological advances in research methodologies currently allow investigators to retrieve an enormous amount of detail regarding any given individual's response to psychotropic medications. Unfortunately, research has not yet been conducted that would establish the cost effectiveness of using these research methodologies in everyday clinical practice and that could perhaps eliminate the need for discussions of pharmacology as it relates to various ethnic groups. Therefore, the nature of the Hispanic response to psychotropic medications must be clarified using extant pharmacological facts.

Beginning with the 1970 census, Mexicans, Central Americans, Cubans, Puerto Ricans, South Americans, and individuals of Spanish descent living in the United States have all been grouped under the umbrella term *Hispanic* (Oboler 1995). Although it is generally perceived that there are significant differences in many sociocultural domains across Hispanic subgroups, what is more important when considering pharmacological response is that genetic variability between subgroups has been clearly demonstrat-

Supported in part by National Institute of Mental Health Research Center on the Psychobiology of Ethnicity Grant no. MH47193.

ed (Vargas-Alarcon et al. 1994). Several genetic mutations in the body's drug-metabolizing–enzyme system have been identified that appear unique to certain ethnic and racial groups and, to a large extent, underlie the differential response to psychotropic medications. Understanding the significance of the genetic variability among Hispanic subgroups, in relationship to the identified ethnic-specific isozymes of the drug-metabolizing enzymes, is important for clinicians. Further refinements can be made in pharmacological treatment of Hispanic patients when clinicians strive also to understand how the Hispanic culture affects pharmacological response. This is especially true for psychotropic medications metabolized by other drug-metabolizing enzymes that are not thought to be under genetic control but that have been shown to be extremely sensitive to environmental factors.

In light of the ongoing demographic shifts in the population of the United States, it is anticipated that American psychiatrists will be routinely involved in the pharmacological treatment of Hispanic patients. In this chapter, we begin by summarizing the data that support genetic variation among Hispanic subgroups. A brief review of the mechanisms involved in the biotransformation of psychoactive compounds follows, with an emphasis on the pharmacogenetics of the cytochrome P450 (CYP) drug-metabolizing–enzyme system as it relates to Hispanics. We then review the literature involving clinical observations of Hispanics receiving psychotropic compounds and anchor this to the existing pharmacological knowledge base. Lastly, recognizing that both doctor and patient exist in a cultural context, we offer some practical guidelines for bridging the cultural gap and optimizing psychopharmacotherapeutic response.

Hispanic Subpopulations: Similar Origins, Divergent Histories

Recorded history, as it relates to the Hispanic story, supports the recent scientific reports of genetic variability among Hispanic subgroups. In brief, all modern-day Hispanics (except those of Spanish descent) are believed to have descended from ancestral Asian and Mongoloid populations. A significant migration of these ancient northeast Siberian people across the Bering Strait is believed to account for the original settlement of North, Central, and South America (Schurr et al. 1990). Except for occasional intertribal warfare, Indians on the North American continent and native peoples in the Caribbean thrived and were probably exposed only to the mutagenic forces inherent in their unique environmental flora and fauna.

The rise in preeminence of the Spanish empire in the late fifteenth and early sixteenth centuries, however, signaled enormous changes for these populations. To continue expanding their economy and power base, Spaniards traveled to West Africa and abducted Africans for use as slaves, as a cheap labor force. These slaves were taken to many Caribbean islands, including Puerto Rico and Cuba, to work on plantations. Slaves were also sent to work in Mexico and in certain countries in Central and South America. In many of the island countries, conquering Spaniards brought diseases that destroyed many indigenous islanders, changing the relative genetic admixture so that it included more African and Caucasian traits. On the North American continent, the Spanish conquest of Mexico in the sixteenth century (Garrity and Gay 1972) resulted in the interbreeding of conquistadores (Caucasian genetic influences) and Latin Amerindians (largely Asian or Mongoloid genetic inheritance).

Through the recent analysis of genetic admixture rates, differences among current-day Hispanics in the amount of genetic material that has been handed down from ancestral Asian, African, and Caucasian populations have been substantiated. Vargas-Alarcon et al. (1994) reported that mestizos in Mexico had admixture rates of 56% Amerindian (largely Asian genetic influence), 4% African, and 40% Caucasian (Spaniard). Hanis et al. (1991) reported similar findings for Mexican Americans, citing 31% Amerindian, 61% Spanish, and 8% black inheritance for this population. Consistent with these reports of strong Amerindian inheritance among Mexican Americans is the fact that diabetes is two to three times more common in Mexican American adults than in whites. This increased prevalence of diabetes among Mexican Americans is currently thought to be due to the presence of genes of Amerindian ancestry (Flegal et al. 1991).

In contrast to the figures for Mexicans and Mexican Americans, the admixture rates for native Puerto Ricans and Cubans are reported to be 46% African, 4% Amerindian, and 50% Spanish (Bortolini et al. 1995; P. A. Fraser et al. 1996). Puerto Ricans and Cubans in the United States manifest African inheritance rates of 37% and 20%, respectively, along with an 18% Amerindian inheritance (Hanis et al. 1991). In addition, analysis of mitochondrial DNA from inhabitants in several South American and Caribbean countries, including Colombia, Jamaica, and Belize, also revealed high levels of West African inheritance (Blank et al. 1995; Monsalve and Hagelberg 1997; Yunis et al. 1994). Because genetic mutations in the body's main drug-metabolizing–enzyme system have been identified as being largely unique to African, Asian, and Spanish populations, these findings of variability in the genetic admixture rates of Mexican Americans and Hispanics of Caribbean descent have pharmacological significance.

Pharmacogenetics and Genetic Polymorphisms of Drug-Metabolizing Enzymes

Pharmacogenetic research has greatly enhanced our understanding of basic pharmacological mechanisms and refined the psychopharmacological treatments available for all patients (Kalow 1992). Researchers in this field have firmly established the following:

1. Four of the most important CYP enzymes—CYP1A2, CYP2D6, CYP2C19, and CYP3A34—are responsible for the metabolism of many commonly used medications such as antibiotics, cardiovascular agents, analgesics, and *psychotropic* medications (Kalow 1992; Nemeroff et al. 1996).
2. Of the four enzymes, only CYP2D6 and CYP2C19 are known to display polymorphic variability; that is, genetic mutations in these enzymes have given rise to different forms of the same enzyme (Gonzalez and Nebert 1990).
3. With respect to CYP2D6 and CYP2C19, gene structure (genotype) largely dictates the functional expression (phenotype) of the enzymes and certain genotypes are more

prevalent among particular ethnic minority groups (Smith and Mendoza 1996).

4. Depending on the exact nature of the mutation present, the different CYP2D6 isozymes exhibit varying degrees of efficiency in the metabolism of substrate; the range includes poor metabolism, slow metabolism, extensive metabolism, and superextensive metabolism (Smith and Mendoza 1996).

5. CYP1A2 and CYP3A4, although not thought to be under genetic control, have exhibited ethnic variation in enzyme activity and appear to be highly sensitive to environmental influences such as diet, pollutants, smoking, and other medicinal compounds (Anderson et al. 1986; Smith and Mendoza 1996).

Polymorphic Variability: Importance of Metabolism Rate

In early pharmacogenetic research, the functional expression (phenotype) of the most important drug-metabolizing enzyme, CYP2D6, was explored. In population-based research, compounds metabolized by the enzyme were administered to subjects and the ratio of parent drug to metabolite was measured. The early data suggested that only two phenotypes existed in any given population: poor metabolizers (PMs) and extensive metabolizers (EMs) (Gonzalez and Nebert 1990). PMs lack a functional form of the enzyme, which often results in absent or extremely slow rates of drug metabolism and potentially toxic blood levels after administration of standard doses. EMs, on the other hand, rapidly metabolize medications and, as a result, may not achieve therapeutic blood levels at standard doses.

There are large gaps in the phenotyping data for Hispanics residing both in- and outside of the United States. No phenotypic analyses have been conducted to date in Puerto Ricans or Cubans; similarly, no data are available for the inhabitants of the majority of Central and South American countries. In 1988, Arias et al. reported CYP2D6 poor-metabolism frequencies of 0% and 5.2%, respectively, among the relatively isolated Cuna and Ngawbe Guaymi tribes of Panama. The former is consistent with the poor-metabolism frequencies identified for many Asian populations, and the latter is similar to Caucasian percentages. It is difficult to make generalizations from these figures, because they represent frequencies for two small, isolated Central American tribes. Interestingly, a commitment to isolation appears to have resulted in the maintenance of genetic homogeneity among the Cuna; their low rate of poor metabolism reflects a predominant Asian inheritance. The Ngawbe Guaymi have allowed a degree of encroachment from the outside world and their poor-metabolism rate reflects a greater European Caucasian admixture. Lam et al. (1991) published preliminary results from a phenotyping study involving 22 Mexican Americans in South Texas that indicated a CYP2D6 poor-metabolism oxidative frequency of 4.4%. Our group recently completed a phenotypic investigation involving 209 Mexican Americans in Southern California. A CYP2D6 poor-metabolism frequency of 2.8% was discovered (Y. Wan, personal communication, July 1999). Lastly, in a study involving 377 healthy volunteers in Spain, Benitez et al. (1988) established that the frequency of poor metabolism in Spanish volunteers was within the 5%–10% range reported for other Caucasian populations (Agundez et al. 1994).

Polymorphic Variability: Mysteries Unveiled Through Gene-Structure Analysis

Although phenotyping different population groups consistently yielded a clear demarcation between PMs and EMs, unanswered questions remained. For example, if the frequency distribution of PMs among Asian populations appeared to be less than 1%, why did Asians seem to need much lower doses and even then experience increased side effects from many psychotropic compounds? A preponderance of EMs would suggest that this population might require increased doses because they would not be expected to receive any benefit from standard doses. The answer to this puzzle was discovered by researchers who focused on genetic analysis of the enzyme structure (genotyping).

With the use of polymerase chain reaction and restriction fragmentation length polymorphism gene-splicing technologies, analysis of the structure of CYP2D6 resulted in identification of two additional phenotypes: slow metabolizers and superextensive metabolizers. CYP2D6 genotyping revealed a particular genetic mutation in Asians, present in approximately 34% of the population, that results in an enzyme with slower metabolic capacities, much slower than those in Caucasian EMs. Before the emergence of genotyping strategies, this 34% (the slow-metabolism frequency distribution) was subsumed under the Asian extensive-metabolizer Abell curve. In a head-to-head comparison with whites, the fact that a full third of Asian EMs are slow metabolizers makes the overall rate of metabolism for that group much slower than the Caucasian extensive-metabolism rate (Bertilsson et al. 1992). This overall slower rate of metabolism explains why many Asian patients require lower doses of psychotropic medications and forces us to recognize that extensive metabolism is a relative term when different populations are being discussed.

Pharmacogenetic Findings in Asians, Africans, and Spaniards: Implications for Today's Hispanics

There are few pharmacogenetic data for Hispanics. As previously stated, not every Hispanic subgroup has been phenotyped. To the best of our knowledge, our research unit is the only one that has reported on the results of CYP2D6 genotyping in Mexican Americans (Mendoza 1996). There are, however, data regarding isozymes that are thought to be fairly specific to Asians, Africans, and Spaniards.

The CYP2D6J or J mutation, which is linked to slow metabolism, occurs at an extremely high rate among Asians: approximately 47%–70% (Yokota et al. 1993). The rate of occurrence is 23% among whites (Armstrong et al. 1994) and 11.6% among Spaniards (Agundez et al. 1994). The CYP2D6Z or Z mutation enzyme is ostensibly responsible for the slowing of enzyme activity in African blacks (Masimirembwa et al. 1996). The allelic frequency of the Z mutation has been estimated to be about 40% among African Zimbabweans, and among African Americans it is 15%–26% (Leathart et al. 1998; K.-M. Lin, personal communication, July 1999).

A CYP2D6 mutation, the *L* mutation, has been isolated in 7% of Spaniards (Agundez et al. 1995) and is associated with an increase in catalytic activity. This increase is due to the fact that multiple copies of the enzyme are present, producing a superextensive metabolizer. Individuals with this mutation often require larger doses to achieve therapeutic plasma levels. Two other population groups, Ethiopians and Saudi Arabians, have been reported to have high rates of superextensive metabolism (29% and 19%, respectively) (Aklillu et al. 1996; McLellan et al. 1997). These two groups trace their origins to the Moors, who centuries ago occupied vast territories in northern Africa. Historical accounts also reveal that the Moors occupied Spain during the Middle Ages. This increased rate of superextensive metabolism among Spaniards, compared with other European whites such as Swedes (of whom less than 1% are superextensive metabolizers), may be accounted for by the Moorish inheritance.

Taken together, these pharmacogenetic data allow for gross estimation of response by modern-day Hispanics to CYP2D6 psychotropic compounds. Hispanics from the Caribbean with admixure rates that reflect a large amount of Asian and African black genetic influence would be expected to have an overall slower rate of metabolism of compounds biotransformed by CYP2D6 compared with Caucasians. This slower rate would be explained by the presence of the *J* and *Z* mutations linked to Asian and African black populations, respectively. Mexicans and Mexican Americans, on the other hand, with a preponderance of Asian and Spaniard genetic inheritance, would be expected to have intermediate-to extensive-metabolism rates, depending on the prevalence of the *J* mutation. Moreover, extremely fast rates of metabolism might be expected among Mexican Americans if the Spaniard *L* mutation is highly prevalent.

Preliminary results from a study our group was conducting of dextromethorphan (a CYP2D6 substrate) metabolism in four ethnic groups in Southern California appear to support some of these assumptions (Mendoza et al., submitted). The frequency distribution of PMs in the Mexican American study sample was 2.8%, midway between that for Asians and whites. The Mexican American cohort exhibited the fastest rate of dextromethorphan metabolism compared with Asian Americans, African Americans, and Caucasians. In this investigation, the relationship of phenotyping to several known CYP2D6 genotypes among the Mexican American subjects was also studied. The allelic frequency of *J1* (mutation in exon 1) in Mexican Americans was 15%, compared with 65% in the Asian American cohort and 26% in Caucasians. The allelic frequency of *J9* (mutation in exon 9) was shown to be 42% in Mexican Americans, 70% in Asian Americans, and 50% in whites. The allelic frequency for the Z mutation was found to be 0.3% in the Mexican American study sample and 15.1% in the black cohort. Lastly, the allelic frequency for the L mutation (gene-duplication mutation) was only 1.9% in Mexican Americans, compared with 0% for all other cohorts. There were no homozygotes identified for the L mutation; however, four heterozygotes were found in the study sample.

One of the more interesting findings of this study rests in the explanation for the faster rate of metabolism in the Mexican American cohort. We had initially hypothesized that this faster rate of metabolism was due to the presence of the L mutation. However, only four heterozygotes for the gene-duplication mutation were identified. Several other factors account for the faster rate of metabolism among the Mexican Americans in the sample: lower penetrance of the J mutation compared with the other groups, complete absence of the Z mutation in the group, and a lower penetrance of the B mutation (which accounts for the majority of PMs among Caucasians) in Mexican Americans than in whites (13% compared with 18%). In comparison with the other three groups studied, our sample of Mexican American subjects had the smallest amount of penetrance of mutant alleles known to code for poor or slow metabolism. This relative protection from poor- and slow-metabolizer alleles appears to explain the overall faster rate of metabolism.

CYP2C19

CYP2C19 has also been shown to exhibit polymorphic variability and is thought to be under primary genetic control (Bertilsson et al. 1989). This enzyme is involved in the metabolism of a number of different psychotropic compounds, such as tricyclic antidepressants (TCAs), barbiturates, citalopram, and diazepam (Bertilsson et al. 1989; Coutts and Urichuk 1999; Kalow 1992; Nemeroff et al. 1996). Although data exist indicating ethnic variability with regard to this isozyme (Smith and Mendoza 1996), these data are not reviewed. In most cases, metabolism of psychotropic compounds by this enzyme is a minor metabolic pathway and/or the drugs metabolized by CYP2C19 are not widely used in psychiatry today.

Cytochrome P450 Enzyme System

In the previous discussion of the CYP2D6 enzyme, genetic control of functional expression of the enzyme was emphasized. The importance of genetics notwithstanding, the pharmacokinetic profile of CYP2D6 substrates can be altered by a number of medicinal compounds and certain dietary substances (Anderson et al. 1986; Kalow 1992). However, when the catalytic activity of two additional CYP enzymes, CYP1A2 and CYP3A4, is considered, the power of non–genetically determined factors to influence metabolism of psychotropic medications is more readily demonstrated.

CYP1A2 has been shown to metabolize theophylline, propranolol, phenacetin, and caffeine, as well as a number of psychotropics, including imipramine, clomipramine, fluvoxamine, clozapine, and olanzapine (Nemeroff et al. 1996; Ring et al. 1996). CYP3A3/4 accounts for more than 50% of the P450 enzymes in the liver and has been found to play a role in the metabolism of cyclosporine, erythromycin, several cardiac drugs (quinidine, verapamil, diltiazem, and nifedipine), antihistamines (terfenadine and astemizole) (Nemeroff et al. 1996), cocaine (Pasanen et al. 1995), and sildenafil (Viagra) (Goldenberg 1998). Among the psychotropics metabolized by CYP3A3/4 are several benzodiazepines, including alprazolam, midazolam, and triazolam; the antidepressants imipramine and nefazodone; and the antipsychotics clozapine, quetiapine, and ziprasidone (Ereshefsky 1996).

CYP1A2 and CYP3A4 do not appear to be under primary genetic control, and therefore no polymorphic variability has been revealed. These enzymes exhibit a striking interindividual variability in the rate of substrate metabolism (Castaneda-Hernandez et al. 1992). This interindividual variability is believed to be due to the inhibition and induction of these enzymes by a host of non–genetically determined factors. For example, the catalytic activity of CYP1A2 is increased by environmental toxins such as the polycyclic aromatic hydrocarbons generated by air pollution, cigarette smoking, and charbroiling of beef (Conney et al. 1977). In addition, indole-containing vegetables such as cabbage and brussels sprouts have been shown to increase the metabolic activity of CYP1A2 (Anderson et al. 1991). Because these enzymes are highly inducible, it is reasonable to expect their catalytic activity to vary substantially across ethnic or cultural groups with divergent dietary habits (Smith and Mendoza 1996).

Dietary Effects on Drug Metabolism

It is becoming increasingly recognized that diet can have a powerful effect on the metabolism of various drugs. Several studies have demonstrated that dietary manipulations significantly alter the pharmacokinetics of many drugs, including certain psychotropic compounds (Anderson et al. 1991; Yang et al. 1992). For example, high-protein diets have been shown to enhance drug metabolism through increased drug oxidation and conjugation (Anderson et al. 1991). In addition, although no similar effect has been well documented in humans, alterations in dietary fat content have resulted in significant changes in the metabolic efficiency of the P450 system in animals (Anderson et al. 1991; Yang et al. 1992).

The relationship between dietary practices, ethnicity, and variability in drug response was first reported by Branch et al. (1978), who compared the rate of antipyrine biotransformation in three study cohorts. The results from this study along with those from two similarly designed follow-up studies (Desai et al. 1980; H. S. Fraser et al. 1979) suggest the following: when members of a population immigrate (especially to an industrialized country) and either abandon or significantly alter the dietary habits practiced in their homeland, they begin to metabolize drugs similarly to the way in which the population of their new country metabolizes them. Although the studies by Branch et al. (1978) did not involve Hispanics, the importance of diet in modulating CYP1A2 and CYP3A4 enzyme activity and the variable of immigration were underscored in these results. By using this knowledge regarding dietary effects on pharmacokinetics along with knowledge of customary dietary practices among Hispanics, physicians can better understand the Hispanic psychopharmacological response.

To illustrate, let us link additional published data regarding certain dietary effects on the CYP3A4 enzyme to some of the known dietary practices among Hispanics. A large concentration of the CYP3A4 enzyme exists in the small intestine. A group of dietary substances known as flavonoids have been demonstrated to influence both CYP1A2 and CYP3A4, with effects including inhibiting intestinal agglomeration of CYP3A4 (Obermeier et al. 1995). In 1984, Waller et al. reported that the metabolism of nifedipine (an antihypertensive) was inhibited by the flavonoid quercetin. This inhibition resulted in an increased bioavailability of nifedipine, along with subsequent increased hypotensive and positive chronotropic effects (Bailey et al. 1991). A similar enhanced response to nifedipine was observed when Mexican subjects were fed a corn-rich diet (Palma-Aguirre et al. 1994). Corn is rich in quercetin and is a dietary staple for many Hispanics. These data should prompt clinicians to consider downwardly adjusting nifedipine doses when treating Hispanics who frequently eat corn and corn tortillas. Similar considerations would seem in order when prescribing certain benzodiazepines to citrus-loving Hispanics. Fuhr (1998) reported that the flavonoid naringin found in grapefruit juice has the capability of inhibiting CYP3A4 in the small intestine. This inhibition resulted in delayed metabolism and enhanced pharmacological effects of several CYP3A4 substrates, including the benzodiazepines triazolam and midazolam.

Concomitant Medications

Psychiatric patients often take multiple psychotropic medications and have medical illnesses that require additional pharmacotherapeutic treatments. Psychiatric practitioners must recognize that administration of multiple medications can alter pharmacokinetic profiles of compounds that are biotransformed by the CYP enzymes. For example, the addition of the popular selective serotonin reuptake inhibitor (SSRI) fluoxetine to a treatment regimen for depression that includes the TCA desipramine has been reported to produce toxic levels of the TCA because of competitive inhibition of CYP2D6 (Dahl et al. 1992). It also appears that in certain cases, use of multiple drugs can transform a known EM into a PM because of competitive inhibition. Llerena et al. (1993) suggested that competitive inhibition was responsible for the 46% rate of poor metabolism observed among drug-treated patients, in contrast to the usual rate of 3%–9% identified in individuals not receiving medication. An extensive discussion of drug-drug interactions and their relationship to the CYP drug-metabolizing–enzyme system is beyond the purview of this chapter. However, a number of reviews have recently been published (Nemeroff et al. 1996; Tanaka and Hisawa 1999). With respect to psychotropic compounds, several are metabolized by more than one enzyme pathway, and clinicians should inform themselves of the major route of metabolism when considering the potential for drug interactions.

Knowledge of the diseases that are prevalent among Hispanics and the medications that are used to treat them allows us to focus on likely interactions. Although Hispanics represent approximately 8.4% of the United States population, 27% of adult and adolescent AIDS cases and 23% of pediatric AIDS cases reported in the country, as of December 1996, occurred in Hispanics (Fernandez et al. 1993; P. Ruiz et al. 1998). HIV is spreading more rapidly in women than in any other group in the United States (Rowe 1998), and most women with AIDS in the United States are either black or Hispanic. Patients in whom HIV infection is diagnosed often develop comorbid psychiatric conditions such as depression or psychosis. As a result, in addition to receiving protease inhibitors such as ritonavir, these patients may also be prescribed adjunctive psychotropic compounds. Because several of these protease inhibitors are potent inhibitors of CYP enzymes, the potential for serious drug interactions exists (Barry et al. 1999; Malaty and Kuper 1999).

Tuberculosis is another medical condition that is highly prevalent in Hispanics (Bloch et al. 1994). In contrast to the CYP inhibitory effects seen with HIV antivirals, treatment with the antituberculin drug rifampin appears to bring about CYP enzyme induction. This enzyme induction by rifampin is thought to account for the lack of response to concurrently prescribed antipsychotics in patients being treated for both psychotic disorders and tuberculosis (Li et al. 1997).

Herbal Preparations

Along with these Western-based treatments, a number of patients, especially Hispanics, use herbal preparations extensively (Eisenberg et al. 1993; Sankury 1983). Contrary to what most physicians believe, many herbal drugs are pharmacologically active and capable of significant interactions with prescribed drugs, both pharmacokinetically and pharmacodynamically (De Smet 1991). For example, several Chinese herbs, including muscone, ginseng, and glycyrrhiza, have been found to have potent stimulating effects on the CYP enzymes. In contrast, oleanolic acid contained in *Sertia mileensis* and *Ligustrum lucidum* substantially inhibits the activities of these enzymes (Liu 1991).

Herbal medications can produce toxicity as a result of their inherent chemical properties. *Datura candida,* which is used to treat the Hispanic culture–specific syndrome susto, contains large amounts of atropine and scopolamine (De Smet 1991). It can cause atropine toxicity and delirium, especially if combined with TCAs or low-potency phenothiazines. The use of *azarcon,* an herbal preparation with a high lead content that is widely used for the treatment of empacho, another Hispanic culture–specific syndrome, has been linked to the deaths of several children in the United States (Mikhail 1994). Pyrrolizidine alkaloids are the metabolic product of the CYP3A4 biotransformation of the Mexican medicinal plant *Packera candidissima,* as well as of another medicinal herb known as comfrey (Bah et al. 1994; Betz et al. 1994). Pyrrolizidine alkaloids have been reported to be hepatotoxic (Bah et al. 1994). Because they represent a product of metabolism, the risk of hepatotoxity should be linked to the rate of metabolism. Hispanics who engage in "traditional" dietary practices that include corn would be expected to be at lower risk of developing this toxicity. Corn inhibits CYP3A4 metabolism, thereby slowing the rate of toxic metabolite production. Although the risks of toxicity associated with self-administration of herbs must be respected, some of the active pharmacological properties of the herbs may also be responsible for their reported effectiveness. For example, several of the components of the traditional herbal preparation *siete azahares,* used by many Hispanics for the treatment of anxiety and depression, are known to have affinities for the γ-aminobutyric acid (GABA) receptor, as do benzodiazepine compounds (Santos et al. 1994).

Clinical Observations

In the last two decades, several clinical studies have focused on Hispanics and their response to psychotropic compounds. These studies are summarized here and the findings are reexamined, taking into account the expanded ethnopsychopharmacological knowledge base outlined earlier.

Tricyclic Antidepressants

In a retrospective review of records of depressed Hispanic and white female outpatients in New York, differences in antidepressant response were noted (Marcos and Cancro 1982). Hispanics (predominantly Puerto Rican) showed comparable positive outcome with only half the dose given Caucasian patients. More Hispanics (78%) than whites (33%) complained of side effects. Furthermore, almost four times as many Hispanics as Caucasians discontinued pharmacotherapy because of side effects (17% vs. 4.8%). Marcos and Cancro (1982) postulated that characteristic TCA side-effect profiles mimicked somatic symptomatology, resulting in rejection of medication or compliance only with reduced-dose treatment by Hispanic patients. They also suggested that pharmacokinetic factors may be important; however, no plasma TCA levels were obtained in the study. Pharmacogenetic research data have demonstrated that TCAs are metabolized predominantly by CYP2D6 and secondarily by CYP2C19. Both of these enzymes are under primary genetic control. As previously reported, the predominance of Asian and African inheritance among Puerto Ricans would result in an overall slower rate of metabolism of CYP2D6 substrates in this Hispanic subpopulation. This slow rate of metabolism could account for the lower doses and increased side effects among the Hispanic patients.

In a prospective study, Escobar and Tuason (1980) examined differences in antidepressant response in patients from Colombia and the United States. Patients in the United States were studied at two different sites, one that predominantly served whites and the other that predominantly served blacks. The efficacy of trazodone was compared with that of imipramine and placebo in patients who met research diagnostic criteria for depression. The Colombian patients were noted to improve more than patients in the United States, regardless of the treatment selected. Whereas no significant differences were found between responses to trazodone and placebo, imipramine had a significantly better effect than did placebo in all three centers. Colombians did report significantly more anticholinergic side effects. The psychotropic compounds used in this research are, again, metabolized by CYP enzymes under primary genetic control. The allele frequency of the Z mutation has been identified as 15%–26% in African Americans (Leathart et al. 1998; K.-M. Lin, personal communication, July 1999). This mutation is known to produce slow metabolism among African blacks and African Americans. In addition, as previously stated, there is a strong West African inheritance among Colombians. The small sample size and the fact that both African Americans and Caucasians were used for the United States comparison group may have worked in concert to eliminate significant differences.

A comparison of various kinetic parameters of nortriptyline metabolism among 10 Hispanic and 10 white nondepressed volunteers was performed by Gaviria et al. (1986) in Chicago. After receiving a single oral dose of nortriptyline (75 mg), blood samples were drawn over a 96-hour period. Although large interindividual differences were discovered in various pharmacokinetic parameters, no statistically significant differences were found between the groups. Gaviria and colleagues (1986) concluded that the lack of differences between groups could possibly be explained by the use of volunteers instead of depressed patients; that is, the disease state itself may serve to alter drug kinetics. Nortriptyline, like trazodone and imipramine, is metabolized primarily by CYP2D6. In this study, the Hispanics studied were Mexican Americans. Several factors could account for the lack of significant differences. First, this was an extremely small study sample. Second, our group has demonstrated a fast rate of metabolism among Mexican Americans owing to a low penetrance of alleles known to code for poor or slow metabolism. It should be remembered that extensive metabolism is a relative term, and Caucasian EMs have also demonstrated fast rates of metabolism in previous studies (Agundez et al. 1995). Large interindividual variation could be seen without the demonstration of significant differences between groups.

Lin et al. (submitted) examined the pharmacokinetics of imipramine and desipramine in 28 African Americans, 33 Asians, 28 Caucasians, and 30 Mexican Americans. The only significant differences in kinetic parameters were noted in the black cohort. African Americans displayed larger areas under the curve for and had higher maximum concentrations of desipramine. This study is concordant with that by Gaviria et al. (1986) in that no significant differences between Caucasian and Mexican American subjects were demonstrated. The increased area under the curve and maximum concentration in the African American group coincide with the slower metabolism seen with populations genetically similar to African blacks and with other reports of slow metabolism in African Americans (Strickland et al. 1991).

Selective Serotonin Reuptake Inhibitors

Alonso et al. (1997) conducted an open-label study of SSRIs in the treatment of depression in 13 Hispanic (Mexican descent) and 13 non-Hispanic female patients. Patients met DSM-III criteria for depression and were treated for 6 weeks with either fluoxetine or paroxetine. Improvement was similar in both groups, but side effects were reported significantly more often by the non-Hispanics. As in many of the clinical studies involving Hispanic populations, the sample size was extremely small. A preponderance of PMs could have been sampled in the non-Hispanic group, which could account for the increased incidence of side effects. As mentioned earlier, the poor-metabolism rate among Caucasians is 5%–10% (Agundez et al. 1994).

Recently, Versiani et al. (1999) conducted a multicenter study involving 157 subjects in whom major depression and comorbid anxiety had been diagnosed. Subjects were randomly assigned to either fluoxetine therapy (20 mg/day) ($n = 77$) or amitriptyline therapy (50–250 mg/day) ($n = 80$). Patients were recruited from seven centers in five countries: Brazil ($n = 52$), Mexico ($n = 36$),

Peru ($n = 28$), Colombia ($n = 23$), and Venezuela ($n = 18$). The ethnicities of the patients were mestizo (44.6%), Caucasian (36.3%), multiracial (5.7%), and other ethnicities (13.3%). The percentage of patients completing the study (82.8% of the entire study population) did not differ significantly across treatment arms; however, twice as many patients receiving amitriptyline (8.8%) as patients receiving fluoxetine (3.9%) stopped treatment because of adverse events. The only statistically significant difference was in improvement of sleep: there was a greater change from baseline to the end of the study in the amitriptyline-treatment group. Otherwise, a favorable treatment response was obtained at a similar rate with both treatments (approximately 74.4%). The mean dose of amitriptyline was 114.1 mg/day, whereas the fluoxetine dose was fixed at 20 mg/day. Approximately 80% of the sample was white or mestizo; mestizos' genetic inheritance resembles that of Mexican Americans. The results of this study are consistent with the results of the study by Alonso et al. (1997), in that no response differences were noted with fluoxetine.

Typical Antipsychotics

Lu et al. (1987) reported findings from a retrospective study of dose and side effects in patients receiving antipsychotic treatment in a San Francisco public sector general hospital. Records of 158 Asian, black, white, and Hispanic inpatients were reviewed. The initial four-way comparison revealed no significant differences between groups in maximum neuroleptic dose, discharge dose, prevalence of extrapyramidal symptoms (EPS), or neuroleptic dose associated with such symptoms. However, when immigrant status was considered, it was found that Asian and Hispanic immigrants received significantly lower mean maximum doses than did patients born in the United States. Environmental and cultural influences such as diet, alcohol, smoking, and exposure to toxins were postulated to explain the observed differences in drug metabolism. Circa 1987, the majority of antipsychotics used to treat psychotic patients were metabolized by CYP2D6; however, the predominant antipsychotic in use, haloperidol, is also metabolized by CYP1A2 and CYP3A4, both of which are sensitive to environmental influences, especially diet and smoking. The explanations put forth by Lu et al. (1987) may well be valid today.

A recent review of medical records of Caucasian, Asian, and Hispanic patients in whom schizophrenia had been diagnosed and who were treated at Elmhurst Hospital Center in New York was conducted to evaluate for variance in dosing and side effects (presence of movement disorders) (Collazo et al. 1996; S. Ruiz et al. 1996). The outpatient portion of the study revealed that with regard to both actual and weight-standardized dosing, Caucasians received significantly larger doses of neuroleptic agents than did Hispanics or Asians. Also, both Hispanic and Asian subjects were prescribed more low-potency medications than were white subjects. In the inpatient portion of the study, significantly larger doses of antipsychotic medication were also prescribed to white patients than to patients in either of the two ethnic minority samples. As in the study by Lu et al. (1987), immigrant subjects (24 of 27 Hispanics and all of the Asian patients) were foreign born, and dietary or other environmental influences may account for the reported differences.

Atypical Antipsychotics

Few data are available regarding treatment with and response to the newer-generation atypical antipsychotic agents among Hispanics. Tran et al. (1998) reported the results from a study of Hispanic patients with psychotic disorders who were switched to olanzapine therapy after developing haloperidol-induced EPS. Although no ethnic differences with respect to dosing were demonstrated, all patients showed dramatic improvement on scales designed to measure both EPS and target symptoms. Reports from Argentina and Chile indicate that psychotic patients from these countries appear to be well treated with clozapine maintenance doses of approximately 300 mg/day (Ramirez 1996). This dose is smaller than the amount used to successfully treat Caucasians in North America (Meltzer et al. 1989). The experience with risperidone in Latin America (Ramirez 1996) appears to be similar to the experience of many practicing psychiatrists in the United States—that is, many patients require doses up to 6 mg/day, whereas another subset responds well to lower doses.

In a recent double-blind, parallel-group, multicenter study in the United States involving inpatients treated with risperidone, Hispanic patients demonstrated a more rapid rate of symptom improvement with risperidone therapy than did non-Hispanic patients (Frackiewicz et al. 1999). Although both Hispanics and non-Hispanics demonstrated improvement from baseline to week 4, the Hispanics improved significantly faster from week 2 through week 4. In this study, Hispanics also had a higher rate of adverse effects, including EPS. The Hispanic cohort consisted primarily of patients from Puerto Rico and the Dominican Republic. These ethnic groups have significant Asian and African black genetic inheritance and, therefore, have links to slower metabolism. This could account for the faster improvement in the Hispanic cohort, along with the increased side effects.

Improving Pharmacological Response: Integrating Culture and Biology

Any conceptual model of pharmacological response must take into account the known pharmacological facts and the cultural contexts in which the doctor and the patient exist. Ethnic minority patients bring to the doctor-patient relationship an assortment of previous experiences with physicians and/or healers, along with a unique set of beliefs and expectations regarding illness and healing. Physicians also draw on their own sociocultural upbringing when entering into treatment alliances with patients. However, there is no denying that physicians' vast medical and pharmacological knowledge base is anchored in Western-based medical concepts. Only recently has the field of psychiatry wavered from its Western-centric stance and validated, in DSM-IV (American Psychiatric Association 1994), the importance of ethnicity and culture in the process of formulating an accurate diagnosis. And with respect to psychopharmacological considerations, only recently has the medical profession acknowledged that dosing schedules have been developed using findings of studies primarily involving Caucasians, with the demonstrated ethnic variability in medication biotransformation being largely ignored.

Although it is reasonable to assume that enhanced patient outcomes might be realized when there is a good match between a patient and a physician (i.e., when the patient and the physician share the same ancestry, cultural heritage, language, and sex) (Bertakis et al. 1995; Holloway et al. 1992; Mischoulon et al. 1998; Peters 1994; Russell 1988), such a match affords no guarantees. Clinicians must constantly strive to bridge the gap between biological and cultural considerations when treating Hispanic patients, in order to accurately prescribe and subsequently assess the clinical efficacy of medications.

Practical Tips

1. Make the Correct Diagnosis

The cornerstone of appropriate pharmacological management is accurate diagnosis. Many psychopharmacotherapeutic failures can be traced to diagnostic error. Unfortunately, making the right diagnosis can prove extremely difficult with Hispanic patients. Results from a 7-year study of changes in diagnosis among hospitalized patients showed that Hispanics in whom an initial diagnosis of schizophrenia was made were more likely than African American and Caucasian subjects to undergo a change in diagnosis during a subsequent hospitalization (Chen et al. 1996). A number of authors have cited difficulties in making diagnoses in ethnic minorities because of the unconventional manner in which these patients categorize and report symptomatology (Guarnaccia et al. 1990; Jenkins 1988; Simmons and Hughes 1985).

The importance of language vis-à-vis diagnosis and psychopharmacological management was underscored in a study by Lawson et al. (1992). Predominantly Spanish-speaking Hispanic patients in a state hospital were interviewed by a research team of Spanish-speaking clinicians using a structured interview. More than 50% of those in whom a diagnosis of schizophrenia had been made were thought, after the interview, to have a major depressive disorder instead. Clinicians must recognize that apparent thought-processing problems may actually be the result of difficulties involved in thinking in one language while talking in another (Marcos 1979) and, in certain cases, that hallucinations are culturally congruent and not necessarily indicative of a psychotic disorder. In the presence of a significant language barrier, a successful psychiatric interview will require the services of either a bilingual mental health practitioner or a mental health practitioner and an interpreter. When an interpreter is needed, the use of a medically trained interpreter is encouraged. If such an interpreter is not available, a member of the patient's family or a bilingual friend may be used, as long as potential limitations, such as the interpreter's investment in a particular outcome, are recognized (Marcos 1979). We suggest that readers review Appendix I of DSM-IV, in which elements of the cultural formulation are outlined, to increase diagnostic accuracy when evaluating Hispanic patients.

2. Obtain Culture-Specific Information and a List of Current Medications

In light of the pharmacogenetic data previously presented, the need to identify the patient's ancestry (e.g., Mexican) seems apparent. These data can aid the physician in making a gross estimation of genetic admixture so that doses can be adjusted as necessary. The ethnicity of both the parents and the grandparents should be determined.

Assessing whether the patient is an immigrant or a first- or second-generation (or later) American is vital. The less acculturated the patient, the more the practitioner should be alerted to the possibility of culture-bound syndromes and, in general, the need to strive diligently for an accurate diagnosis. In addition, the less acculturated the patient, the greater is the likelihood of concomitant use of alternative healing.

Every psychiatric assessment must include an inquiry into the medical history and the current use of prescribed medications. The drugs' pharmacokinetic profiles and enzymatic route of biotransformation, if known, must be factored into the selection of an appropriate psychotropic medication, as well as the decision about a need for dose adjustments. The clinician should also determine whether the patient has visited *curanderos* (a spiritual or mystic healer) or spiritualists and, if the patient has done so, determine the nature of the treatments given. Questions regarding the use of medicinal teas should be asked. In our experience, a significant proportion of slightly to moderately acculturated Hispanic women drink medicinal teas such as *té de siete azahares, té de tila,* and *té de valeria* on a regular basis. Also, over-the-counter natural or holistic medicinal preparations are in widespread use across America today. Frank questioning regarding their use is important, and the clinician should request that the patient bring in any pill bottles. The lists of ingredients should be scrutinized for possible toxic substances.

In addition to questions about the use of teas and the like, a brief inventory of the food commonly eaten by Hispanics should be part of the assessment. Specifically, the frequency of ingestion of corn, corn tortillas, and grapefruit juice, as well as the frequency of charbroiling, can be useful when choosing psychotropic compounds or making dosing adjustments (especially when selecting medications metabolized by CYP1A2 or CYP3A4).

3. Provide Practical Medication Education

In our experience, asking about the previous use of compounds such as acetaminophen, salicylic acid, and antibiotics allows the psychiatrist to gain an understanding of the extent of the patient's exposure to and expectations regarding Western-based medications. In addition, it serves as a transition to educating the patient about the differences in the mechanisms of actions of psychotropic medications and, especially, the length of time needed to achieve beneficial effects. Although this strategy can prove extremely useful when initiating medication therapy, emphasizing the chronic nature of chronic medical and psychiatric illnesses will assist in maintaining long-term compliance. Asking whether the patient knows of anyone with chronic medical conditions such as diabetes, seizure disorders, or heart problems and highlighting the importance of long-term pharmacological treatment for such conditions allow the practitioner to make analogies with chronic mental illness and the need for long-term treatment with psychotropics. These concepts should be explained using grade school–level vocabulary, and the patient should be asked to express his or her understanding of the explanation to avoid confusion.

4. Assess Adherence

It is estimated that more than 50% of patients do not adhere to the treatments prescribed by their physicians (Sackett and Haynes 1976). Additional reports (Diaz et al. 1998; Kinzie et al. 1987) indicate that noncompliance is a substantial problem among ethnic minority patients and that a large gap exists between the subjective estimation of medication compliance and the objective evidence of the same. Lastly, studies focusing on predictors of adherence have found that the doctor-patient relationship, encompassing communication regarding drug actions and side effects, plays a crucial role in compliance (Stimson 1974; Svarstad 1976; Zola 1973). Therefore, detailed questioning and monitoring of blood levels are recommended to maximize medication compliance.

Simply asking "Are you taking your medication?" and receiving an affirmative answer do not guarantee adherence with drug therapy. A more detailed set of questions regarding the taking of medications often yields more useful information. For example, patients should be asked exactly how they are taking their medications (how many times a day, what times during the day, and how many pills at what time). Also, patients should be requested to bring in the pill bottles and actually count the pills left. If there appears to be confusion, written instructions in Spanish should be provided.

Quantifying blood levels of those compounds for which assays are available is an easy and reliable method to ensure compliance and assess metabolic status. Reliable assays are currently available for compounds such as nortriptyline, clozapine, olanzapine, risperidone, and all the mood stabilizers.

5. Take Into Account the Patient's Pharmacy Benefit Package

In both the public and private health care sectors, the influence of managed care has led to the development of pharmacy benefit packages for patients that limit pharmacotherapeutic selection. More traditional and older-generation antipsychotics and antidepressants may be preferred because of their reduced per-pill costs. Such clinically irrational influences can adversely affect prescribing practice and may have long-term consequences in the form of suboptimal or negative outcomes. Physicians must remain staunch advocates for their patients and secure approval (despite the paperwork involved with treatment-authorization requests) for a drug selection that is guided by clinical indicators and not by a one-size-fits-all formulary.

6. Consider Polypharmacotherapeutic Approaches

The future of psychopharmacotherapy may include creative dietary or other pharmacological manipulations of the CYP enzyme system to achieve a positive treatment response. Recently, it was demonstrated that levels of cyclosporine (an expensive immunosuppressive agent) were dramatically increased in patients who were concomitantly administered grapefruit juice (Hollander et al. 1995). In other studies, paroxetine and fluoxetine were used to raise desipramine levels in superextensive metabolizers who were nonresponsive to standard doses (Kraus et al. 1996). Also, the authors used fluvoxamine to augment olanzapine and clozapine concentrations when a lack of response was obtained at standard or upper-level doses. Because per-pill costs of many of today's newer-generation psychoactive compounds often prove prohibitive, use of dietary and pharmacological CYP inhibitors could have significant pharmacoeconomic implications.

Conclusion

There are an estimated 22 million Hispanics in the United States: 13.5 million are of Mexican descent, and 2.5 million are of Puerto Rican, 1 million are of Cuban, and 5 million are of Central and South American descent (Oboler 1995). Although these groups share certain sociocultural features, it is clear, given differences in pharmacological response, that these groups cannot be considered together. Recorded history reveals nuances in their unfolding stories, and science, at the level of the gene, reflects their distinctiveness. Unfortunately, although science and technology can currently supply impressive detail regarding how a given individual will metabolize psychotropic compounds, ethnic and subgroup comparisons must still be made.

Findings from two separate lines of research can be linked to formulate an understanding of how Hispanic subgroups might metabolize psychotropic medications that are handled by the CYP enzyme CYP2D6. First, researchers in the field of pharmacogenetics have identified ethnic-specific mutations of CYP2D6 in Asians, African blacks, and Spaniards. Mutations in these populations hold significance because they represent the genetic inheritance of modern-day Hispanics (excluding those of Spanish descent). Second, researchers focusing on genetic admixture rates for various populations have demonstrated differences in the relative inheritance of genetic material from the Hispanic ancestral groups just identified. Caribbean Hispanics (Hispanics of Cuban or Puerto Rican descent) appear to have a substantial amount of African black and Asian inheritance, whereas Mexican Americans and Mexican mestizos have primarily Spanish and Asian inheritance. These differences in the relative amounts of genetic influence can be traced to early slave trading, in the case of Caribbean Hispanics, and the conquest of Mexico by Spaniards, in the case of Mexican mestizos and Mexican Americans.

Because the ethnic-specific mutations in Asians, African blacks, and Spaniards are directly associated with varying degrees of CYP2D6 enzyme efficiency, the genetic admixture data can be used to formulate an idea of the rate of metabolism. For example, because Asian and African black populations have a high rate of occurrence of mutations coding slow-metabolizer status, one might anticipate Hispanics of Cuban or Puerto Rican descent to have similar pharmacokinetic profiles. Side effects might be experienced at standard doses, and clinicians should consider slow titrations and the need for lower doses to maximize compliance when prescribing medications.

Similarly, Spaniards have been shown to have a large penetrance of a mutation that brings about superextensive metabolism. Because Mexican Americans have a disproportionately large amount of Spanish genetic inheritance, faster rates of metabolism might be expected, depending on the degree of penetrance of this mutation. Alternatively, as our research group showed (Mendoza et al., submitted), faster metabolism among Mexican Americans may be due to the *absence* of mutant alleles coding for poor and slow metabolism, stemming from the group's unique genetic admixture. Although these represent preliminary and rough guidelines, a close inspection of the reports of clinical studies featuring Hispanics and the administration of CYP2D6 psychotropic substrates reveals consistency with our assertions.

In contrast to CYP2D6, CYP1A2 and CYP3A4 are not under genetic control but are extremely sensitive to environmental influences such as diet, toxins, and smoking. Drug-drug and drug-diet interactions have been shown to be the result of the ability of certain medications and dietary supplements to act as inducers and inhibitors of the drug-metabolizing enzymes, including CYP2D6. Food items such as corn, grapefruit juice, and *carne asada* (charbroiled beef), usually featured in the Hispanic diet, have been demonstrated to alter the efficiency of CYP1A2 and CYP3A4. In addition, with the tremendous growth of alternative medicine in the past few years, the general public has been given free access to a host of natural and holistic compounds. The use of herbs and alternative medications is widespread among Hispanics, and this use can result in both toxicity as well as modulation of the drug-metabolizing enzymes.

Because the prescription and subsequent use of medications is shrouded in symbolism and social meaning, it is reasonable to expect that culture will exert powerful influences on pharmacological response. The clinician faces a series of obstacles when evaluating a Hispanic patient. Formulation of a diagnosis often proves extremely difficult, especially when the patient is unacculturated and language and other communication barriers are manifest. There are a number of adjustments psychiatrists can make, however, to maximize diagnostic accuracy and subsequent medication compliance.

Striving to understand the patient's previous experiences with Western-based medications and comparing these experiences (in simple terms) with what is necessary and can be expected with psychotropic therapy can minimize confusion. Practical and direct questioning aimed at getting the patient to restate instructions and to detail the use of alternative healing practices and customary dietary intake is prudent. Probing to assess compliance accurately and monitoring blood levels, when possible, are extremely useful when the physician encounters side effects and suboptimal outcomes. Last, being apprised of pharmacogenetic research findings and the emerging drug-interaction literature is mandatory so that the clinician can adjust dosing and/or add inhibitors to the patient's treatment as needed. Clearly, integrating pharmacological facts with cultural considerations affords the prescribing psychiatrist the best opportunity for a positive psychopharmacotherapeutic outcome.

The data regarding Hispanics and psychopharmacology remain extremely scarce. To date, no phenotyping and genotyping data exist for Hispanics of Puerto Rican or Cuban descent. Data are lacking that reflect experiences among Hispanics with many of the newer antidepressants, including pharmacokinetic profiling and clinical efficacy data. To the best of our knowledge, no reports have been published concerning the use of mood stabilizers by Hispanics with cycling affective illness. Last, no head-to-head comparison of pharmacological response across all Hispanic subgroups has been conducted. We reviewed the Hispanic psychopharmacology literature approximately 10 years ago (Mendoza et al. 1991). Afforded this opportunity to take a second, closer look, we have found that the field has moved forward but that there is much we still do not know.

References

Agundez JA, Martinez C, Ledesma MC, et al: Genetic basis for differences in debrisoquin polymorphism between a Spanish and other white populations. Clin Pharmacol Ther 55:412–417, 1994

Agundez JA, Ledesma MC, Ladero JM, et al: Prevalence of CYP2D6 gene duplication and its repercussion on the oxidative phenotype in a white population. Clin Pharmacol Ther 57:265–269, 1995

Aklillu E, Persson I, Bertilsson L, et al: Frequent distribution of ultrarapid metabolizers of debrisoquine in an Ethiopian population carrying duplicated and multiduplicated functional CYP2D6 alleles. J Pharmacol Exp Ther 278:441–446, 1996

Alonso M, Val E, Rapaport MH: An open-label study of SSRI treatment in depressed Hispanic and non-Hispanic women (letter). J Clin Psychiatry 58:31, 1997

American Psychiatric Association: Diagnostic and Statistical Manual of Mental Disorders, 3rd Edition. Washington, DC, American Psychiatric Association, 1980

American Psychiatric Association: Diagnostic and Statistical Manual of Mental Disorders, 4th Edition. Washington, DC, American Psychiatric Association, 1994

Anderson KE, Conney AH, Kappas A: Nutrition as an environmental influence on chemical metabolism in man: ethnic differences in reactions to drugs and xenobiotics. Prog Clin Biol Res 214:39–54, 1986

Anderson KE, McCleery RB, Vesell ES, et al: Diet and cimetidine induce comparable changes in theophylline metabolism in normal subjects. Hepatology 13:941–946, 1991

Arias TD, Inaba T, Cooke RG, et al: A preliminary note on the transient polymorphic oxidation of sparteine in the Ngawbe Guaymi Amerindians: a case of genetic divergence with tentative phylogenetic time frame for the pathway. Clin Pharmacol Ther 44:343–352, 1988

Armstrong M, Fairbrother K, Idle JR, et al: The cytochrome P450 CYP2D6 allelic variant *CYP2D6J* and related polymorphisms in a European population. Pharmacogenetics 4:73–81, 1994

Bah M, Bye R, Pereda-Miranda R: Hepatotoxic pyrrolizidine alkaloids in the Mexican medicinal plant *Packera candidissima* (Asteraceae: Senecioneae). J Ethnopharmacol 43:19–30, 1994

Bailey DG, Spence JD, Munoz C, et al: Interaction of citrus juices with felodipine and nifedipine. Lancet 337:268–269, 1991

Barry M, Mulcahy F, Merry C, et al: Pharmacokinetics and potential interactions amongst antiretroviral agents used to treat patients with HIV infection. Clin Pharmacokinet 36:289–304, 1999

Benitez J, Llerena A, Cobaleda J: Debrisoquin oxidation polymorphism in a Spanish population. Clin Pharmacol Ther 44:74–77, 1988

Bertakis KD, Helms LJ, Callahan EJ, et al: The influence of gender on physician practice style. Med Care 33:407–416, 1995

Bertilsson L, Henthorn TK, Sanz E, et al: Importance of genetic factors in the regulation of diazepam metabolism: relationship to *S*-mephenytoin, but not debrisoquin, hydroxylation phenotype. Clin Pharmacol Ther 45:348–355, 1989

Bertilsson L, Lou YQ, Du YL, et al: Pronounced differences between native Chinese and Swedish populations in the polymorphic hydroxylations of debrisoquin and *S*-mephenytoin. Clin Pharmacol Ther 51:388–397, 1992

Betz JM, Eppley RM, Taylor WC, et al: Determination of pyrrolizidine alkaloids in commercial comfrey products (*Symphytum* sp.). J Pharm Sci 83:649–653, 1994

Blank M, Blank A, King S, et al: Distribution of HLA and haplotypes of Colombian and Jamaican black populations. Tissue Antigens 45:111–116, 1995

Bloch AB, Cauthen GM, Onorato IM, et al: Nationwide survey of drug-resistant tuberculosis in the United States. JAMA 271:665–671, 1994

Bortolini MC, Weimer T de A, Salzano FM, et al: Evolutionary relationships between black South American and African populations. Hum Biol 67:547–559, 1995

Branch RA, Smith SY, Homeida M: Racial differences in drug metabolizing ability: a study with antipyrine in the Sudan. Clin Pharmacol Ther 24:283–286, 1978

Castaneda-Hernandez G, Hoyo-Vadillo C, Palma-Aguirre A, et al: Pharmacokinetics of oral nifedipine in different populations. J Clin Pharmacol 32:140–145, 1992

Chen YR, Swann AC, Burt DB: Stability of diagnosis in schizophrenia. Am J Psychiatry 153:682–686, 1996

Collazo Y, Tam R, Sramek J, et al: Neuroleptic dosing in Hispanic and Asian inpatients with schizophrenia. Mt Sinai J Med 63:310–313, 1996

Conney AH, Pantuck EJ, Hsiao KC, et al: Regulation of drug metabolism in man by environmental chemicals and diet. Federation Proceedings 36:1647–1652, 1977

Coutts RT, Urichuk LJ: Polymorphic cytochromes P450 and drugs used in psychiatry. Cell Mol Neurobiol 19:325–354, 1999

Dahl ML, Johansson I, Palmertz MP, et al: Analysis of the *CYP2D6* gene in relation to debrisoquin and desipramine hydroxylation in a Swedish population. Clin Pharmacol Ther 51:12–17, 1992

Desai, NK, Sheth UK, Mucklow JC: Antipyrine clearance in Indian villagers. Br J Clin Pharmacol 9:387–394, 1980

De Smet PA: Is there any danger in using traditional remedies? J Ethnopharmacol 32:43–50, 1991

Diaz E, Barry V, Pearsall HR, et al: Comparing subjective medication adherence with an objective method. Presented at the annual meeting of the American Psychiatric Association, Toronto, ON, Canada, May–June 1998

Eisenberg DM, Kessler RC, Foster C, et al: Unconventional medicine in the United States: prevalence, costs, and patterns of use. N Engl J Med 328:246–252, 1993

Ereshefsky L: Pharmacokinetics and drug interactions: update for new antipsychotics. J Clin Psychiatry 57(suppl 11):12–25, 1996

Escobar JI, Tuason VB: Antidepressant agents: a cross cultural study. Psychopharmacol Bull 16:49–52, 1980

Fernandez F, Ruiz P, Bing EG: The mental health impact of AIDS on ethnic minorities, in Culture, Ethnicity, and Mental Illness. Edited by Gaw AC. Washington, DC, American Psychiatric Press, 1993, pp 573–586

Flegal KM, Ezzatti TM, Harris MI, et al: Prevalence of Diabetes in Mexican Americans, Cubans, and Puerto Ricans from the Hispanic Health and Nutrition Examination Survey, 1982–1984. Diabetes Care 14:628–638, 1991

Frackiewicz E, Sramek J, Collazo Y, et al: Risperidone in the treatment of Hispanic schizophrenic inpatients, in Cross Cultural Psychiatry. Edited by Herrera JM, Lawson WB, Sramek JJ. New York, Wiley, 1999, pp 183–192

Fraser HS, Mucklow JC, Bulpitt CJ, et al: Environmental factors affecting antipyrine metabolism in London factory and office workers. Br J Clin Pharmacol 7:237–243, 1979

Fraser PA, Yunis EJ, Alper CA: Excess admixture proportion of extended major histocompatibility complex haplotypes of Caucasian origin among rheumatoid arthritis associated haplotypes in African Americans and Afro-Caribbeans. Ethnicity and Health 1(2):153–159, 1996

Fuhr U: Drug interactions with grapefruit juice: extent, probable mechanism and clinical relevance. Drug Saf 18:251–272, 1998

Garrity JA, Gay PE (eds): The Columbia History of the World. New York, Harper & Row, 1972

Gaviria M, Gil AA, Javaid JI: Nortriptyline kinetics in Hispanic and Anglo subjects. J Clin Psychopharmacol 6:227–231, 1986

Goldenberg MM: Safety and efficacy of sildenafil citrate in the treatment of male erectile dysfunction. Clin Ther 20:1033–1048, 1998

Gonzalez FJ, Nebert DW: Evolution of the P450 gene superfamily: animal-plant "warfare," molecular drive and human genetic differences in drug oxidation. Trends Genet 6:182–186, 1990

Guarnaccia PJ, Good BJ, Kleinman A: A critical review of epidemiological studies of Puerto Rican mental health. Am J Psychiatry 147:1449–1456, 1990

Hanis CL, Hewett-Emmett D, Bertin TK, et al: Origins of U.S. Hispanics: implications for diabetes. Diabetes Care 14:618–627, 1991

Hollander AA, van Rooij J, Lentjes GW, et al: The effect of grapefruit juice on cyclosporine and prednisone metabolism in transplant patients. Clin Pharmacol Ther 57:318–324, 1995

Holloway RL, Rogers JC, Gershenhorn SL: Differences between patient and physician perceptions of predicted compliance. Fam Pract 9:318–322, 1992

Jenkins JH: Conceptions of schizophrenia as a problem of nerves: a cross-cultural comparison of Mexican-Americans and Anglo-Americans. Soc Sci Med 26:1233–1243, 1988

Kalow W: Pharmacogenetics of Drug Metabolism. New York, Pergamon, 1992

Kinzie JD, Leung P, Boehnlein J, et al: Tricyclic antidepressant plasma levels in Indochinese refugees: clinical and cultural implications. J Nerv Ment Dis 175:480–485, 1987

Kraus RP, Diaz P, McEachran A: Managing rapid metabolizers of antidepressants. Depress Anxiety 4:320–327, 1996

Lam Y, Castro D, Dunn J: Drug metabolizing capacity in Mexican Americans (abstract). Clin Pharmacol Ther 49:159, 1991

Lawson W, Herrera J, Costa J: The dexamethasone suppression test as an adjunct in diagnosing depression. J Assoc Acad Minor Phys 3:17–19, 1992

Leathart JB, London SJ, Steward A: CYP2D6 phenotype-genotype relationships in African Americans and Caucasians in Los Angeles. Pharmacogenetics 8:529–541, 1998

Li AP, Reith MK, Rasmussen A, et al: Primary human hepatocytes as a tool for the evaluation of structure-activity relationship in cytochrome P450 induction potential of xenobiotics: evaluation of rifampin, rifapentine and rifabutin. Chem Biol Interact 107:17–30, 1997

Lin K-M, Poland RE, Nuccio I, et al: Ethnicity and imipramine response: I. pharmacokinetic and pharmacogenetic influences. Submitted for publication

Liu G: Effects of some compounds isolated from Chinese medicinal herbs on hepatic microsomal cytochrome P-450 and their potential biological consequences. Drug Metab Rev 23:439–465, 1991

Llerena A, Herraiz AG, Cobaleda J, et al: Debrisoquin and mephenytoin hydroxylation phenotypes and CYP2D6 genotype in patients treated with neuroleptic and antidepressant agents. Clin Pharmacol Ther 54:606–611, 1993

Lu FG, Chien C-P, Heming G, et al: Ethnicity and neuroleptic drug dosage. Paper presented at the annual meeting of the American Psychiatric Association, Chicago, IL, May 1987

Malaty LI, Kuper JJ: Drug interactions of HIV protease inhibitors. Drug Saf 20:147–169, 1999

Marcos LR: Effects of interpreters on the evaluation of psychopathology in non-English-speaking patients. Am J Psychiatry 136:171–174, 1979

Marcos LR, Cancro R: Pharmacotherapy of Hispanic depressed patients: clinical observations. Am J Psychother 36:505–513, 1982

Masimirembwa CM, Hasler J, Bertilssons L, et al: Phenotype and genotype analysis of debrisoquine hydroxylase (CYP2D6) in a black Zimbabwean population: reduced enzyme activity and evaluation of metabolic correlation of CYP2D6 probe drugs. Eur J Clin Pharmacol 51(2): 117–122, 1996

McLellan RA, Oscarson M, Seidegard J, et al: Frequent occurrence of CYP2D6 gene duplication in Saudi Arabians. Pharmacogenetics 7: 187–191, 1997

Mendoza R, Wan Y, Poland RE, et al: CYP2D6 polymorphism in a Mexican American population: relationship between genotyping and phenotyping. Submitted for publication

Meltzer HY, Alphs L, Bastani B, et al: One year outcome study of clozapine in treatment resistant schizophrenia. Paper presented at the 8th World Congress of Psychiatry, Athens, October 1989

Mendoza R: CYP2D6 genotype in Mexican Americans. Paper presented at the annual meeting of the American Psychiatric Association, New York, May 1996

Mendoza R, Smith MW, Poland RE, et al: Ethnic psychopharmacology: the Hispanic and Native American perspective. Psychopharmacol Bull 27:449–461, 1991

Mikhail BI: Hispanic mothers' beliefs and practices regarding selected children's health problems. West J Nurs Res 16:623–638, 1994

Mischoulon D, Lagomasino IT, Harmon C: Psychotic depression in a Hispanic population: diagnostic dilemmas and implications for treatment. Paper presented at the annual meeting of the American Psychiatric Association, Toronto, ON, Canada, May–June 1998

Monsalve MV, Hagelberg E: Mitochondrial DNA polymorphisms in Carib people of Belize. Proc R Soc Lond B Biol Sci 264:1217–1224, 1997

Nemeroff CB, DeVane CL, Pollock BG: Newer antidepressants and the cytochrome P450 system. Am J Psychiatry 153:311–320, 1996

Obermeier MT, White RE, Yang CS: Effects of bioflavonoids on hepatic P450 activities. Xenobiotica 25:575–584, 1995

Oboler S: Ethnic Labels, Latino Lives: Identity and the Politics of (Re)Presentation in the United States. Minneapolis, MN, University of Minnesota Press, 1995

Palma-Aguirre JA, Nava Rangel J, Hoyo-Vadillo C, et al: Influence of Mexican diet on nifedipine pharmacodynamics in healthy volunteers. Proc West Pharmacol Soc 37:85–86, 1994

Pasanen M, Pellinen P, Stenback F, et al: The role of CYP enzymes in cocaine-induced liver damage. Arch Toxicol 69:287–290, 1995

Peters RM: Matching physician practice style to patient informational issues and decision making preferences. Arch Fam Med 3:760–763, 1994

Ramirez L: Ethnicity and psychopharmacology in Latin America. Mt Sinai J Med 63:330–331, 1996

Ring BJ, Catlow J, Lindsay TJ, et al: Identification of the human cytochromes P450 responsible for the in vitro formation of the major oxidative metabolites of the antipsychotic agent olanzapine. J Pharmacol Exp Ther 276:658–666, 1996

Rowe C: Special issues of women with AIDS and HIV disease. Paper presented at the annual meeting of the American Psychiatric Association, Toronto, ON, Canada, May–June 1998

Ruiz P, Munoz RA, Dominguez MN, et al: Treatment and prevention. Paper presented at the annual meeting of the American Psychiatric Association, Toronto, ON, Canada, May–June 1998

Ruiz S, Chu P, Sramek J, et al: Neuroleptic dosing in Asian and Hispanic outpatients with schizophrenia. Mt Sinai J Med 63:306–309, 1996

Russell D: Language and psychotherapy: the influence of nonstandard English in clinical practice, in Clinical Guidelines in Cross-Cultural Mental Health (Wiley Series in General and Clinical Psychiatry). Edited by Comas-Diaz L, Griffith E. New York, Wiley, 1988, pp 33–68

Sackett DL, Haynes RB (eds): Compliance With Therapeutic Regimens. Baltimore, MD, Johns Hopkins University Press, 1976

Sankury T: Lead poisoning from Mexican folk remedies—California (letter). JAMA 250:3149, 1983

Santos MS, Ferreira F, Faro C, et al: The amount of GABA present in aqueous extracts of valerian is sufficient to account for [3H]GABA release in synaptosomes. Planta Med 60:475–476, 1994

Schurr TG, Ballinger SW, Gan YY, et al: Amerindian mitochondrial DNAs have rare Asian mutations at high frequencies, suggesting they derived from four primary maternal lineages. Am J Hum Genet 46:613–623, 1990

Simmons R, Hughes C: The Culture Bound Syndromes: Folk Illnesses of Psychiatric and Anthropological Interest. Boston, Reidel, 1985

Smith M, Mendoza R: Ethnicity and pharmacogenetics. Mt Sinai J Med 63:285–290, 1996

Stimson GV: Obeying doctor's orders: a view from the other side. Soc Sci Med 8:97–104, 1974

Strickland TL, Rangananth V, Lin KM, et al: Psychopharmacologic considerations in the treatment of black American populations. Psychopharmacol Bull 27:441–448, 1991

Svarstad B: Physician-patient communication and patient conformity with medical advice, in The Growth of Bureaucratic Medicine: An Inquiry Into the Dynamics of Patient Behavior and the Organization of Medical Care. Edited by Mechanic D. New York, Wiley, 1976, pp 220–238

Tanaka E, Hisawa S: Clinically significant pharmacokinetic drug interactions with psychoactive drugs: antidepressants and antipsychotics and the cytochrome P450 system. J Clin Pharm Ther 24:7–16, 1999

Tran P, Tohen M, Mazzoti G, et al: Switching psychotic patients with symptomatic extrapyramidal symptoms from haloperidol to olanzapine: results of a multi-center, collaborative trial in Latin America. Paper presented at the annual meeting of the American Psychiatric Association, Toronto, ON, Canada, May–June 1998

Vargas-Alarcon G, Garcia A, Bahena S, et al: HLA-B alleles and complotypes in Mexican patients with seronegative spondyloarthropathies. Ann Rheum Dis 53:755–758, 1994

Versiani M, Ontiveros A, Mazzotti G, et al: Fluoxetine versus amitriptyline in the treatment of major depression with associated anxiety (anxious depression): a double-blind comparison, in Cross Cultural Psychiatry. Edited by Herrera JM, Lawson WB, Sramek JJ. New York, Wiley, 1999, pp 249–258

Waller DG, Renwick AG, Gruchy BS, et al: The first pass metabolism of nifedipine in man. Br J Clin Pharmacol 18:951–954, 1984

Yang CS, Brady JF, Hong JY: Dietary effects on cytochromes P450, xenobiotic metabolism, and toxicity. FASEB J 6:737–744, 1992

Yokota H, Tamura S, Furuya H, et al: Evidence for a new variant CYP2D6 allele CYP2D6J in a Japanese population associated with lower in vivo rates of sparteine metabolism. Pharmacogenetics 3:256–263, 1993

Yunis J, Ossa H, Salazar M, et al: Major histocompatibility complex class II alleles and haplotypes and blood groups of four Amerindian tribes of northern Colombia. Hum Immunol 41:248–258, 1994

Zola IK: Pathways to the doctor—from person to patient. Soc Sci Med 7:677–684, 1973

Chapter 4

Ethnopsychopharmacology for Asians

Edmond H. Pi, M.D.
Gregory E. Gray, M.D., Ph.D.

There has been growing evidence that ethnicity is an important factor in an individual's pharmacological response to psychotropic medications. Interest in this area has further increased as a result of the discovery of genetic polymorphism in enzyme systems responsible for metabolizing most of the psychotropic medications (Pi and Gray 1998; Sramek and Pi 1999). However, studies have often yielded conflicting findings, and many questions regarding the transcultural aspects of psychotropic medications remain unanswered (Pi and Gray 1998).

The most studied ethnic differences in transcultural psychopharmacology have been those between Caucasian and Asian populations. In this chapter, we review pharmacokinetics, pharmacodynamics, and sociocultural influences on drug response in Asians, focusing on the major classes of psychotropic medications.

Pharmacogenetics

Pharmacogenetics is the study of the relationship between an individual's genotype and his or her ability to metabolize particular pharmacological compounds (Linder et al. 1997). An individual's pharmacogenetic profile can influence both the pharmacokinetics and the pharmacodynamics of a given medication.

Pharmacokinetics

Pharmacokinetics is concerned with the way in which the body handles drugs, including the absorption, distribution, metabolism, and excretion of drugs. There are a number of well-studied pharmacogenetic differences leading to interindividual as well as interethnic differences in rates of drug metabolism. One of the best known of these involves ethanol metabolism (Agarwal and Goedde 1990). Approximately 50% of East Asians lack the active form of the enzyme aldehyde dehydrogenase because of a single amino acid substitution. This enzyme deficiency results in the accumulation of acetaldehyde and the "flushing" response (facial flushing and palpitations). In addition, 85%–90% of Chinese and other East Asians have an "atypical" alcohol dehydrogenase isozyme with greater capacity to convert alcohol into acetaldehyde, further contributing to the flushing reaction.

Acetylation of drugs is also associated with genetically determined interindividual and interethnic differences. Differences in isoniazid toxicity between Asians and Caucasians are due to acetylation enzyme polymorphism. The majority (78%–93%) of Chinese and East Asians are fast acetylators, whereas only 50% of whites and African Americans are fast acetylators (Weber 1987). This is clinically important, because several psychoactive compounds (e.g., caffeine, clonazepam, nitrazepam, and phenelzine) are metabolized through acetylation (Sjoqvist et al. 1997).

The activities of the conjugating enzymes (transferases) are also genetically determined, but these activities can be induced by various environmental factors such as alcohol, coffee, oral contraceptives, diet, and tobacco as well (Mucklow et al. 1980). An example of interethnic differences in conjugation can be seen in the clearance of acetaminophen (85%–90% excreted after glucuronide or sulfate conjugation), which is 20% slower in Asians than in Europeans.

The cytochrome P450 (CYP) system is the group of enzymes of most interest to psychiatrists. These enzymes show considerable genetic variation, and certain isozymes can be induced by specific substrates such as phenobarbital, ethanol, and steroids. They can also be inhibited by various medications that are potent competitive inhibitors of the enzymes (e.g., cimetidine and ketoconazole).

In recent years, considerable information about this group of enzymes and its genetic variation has become available (Richelson 1997; Sjoqvist et al. 1997). The CYP enzymes show genetic polymorphism, with the result that individuals are classified as extensive metabolizers (EMs), poor metabolizers (PMs), or slow metabolizers (SMs), depending on whether they carry genetic mutations that alter the amino acid structure and activity of the enzymes (Gonzalez 1992; Kalow 1991). Differences in rates of psychotropic medication metabolism are related to the genetic polymorphism and subsequent functional expression of the CYP enzymes, particularly CYP2D6 and CYP2C19.

CYP2D6 (debrisoquin hydroxylase) is involved in the metabolism of a large number of psychotropic medications, including most antipsychotics, tricyclic antidepressants (TCAs), selective serotonin reuptake inhibitors (SSRIs), venlafaxine, amphetamines, and propranolol (Pi and Gray 1998; Richelson 1997). The proportion of PMs differs in different ethnic groups. Among Caucasians, 5%–10% are PMs, whereas the proportion of Asians who are PMs is 1%–6% (Edeki 1996; Pi and Gray 1998; Richelson 1997; Sjoqvist et al. 1997). Among the majority of the population with adequate CYP2D6 activity (EMs), there also exists considerable variation in the degree of activity because of genetic polymorphism (Richelson 1997). There are at least nine mutant forms of the enzyme (Kroemer and Eichelbaum 1995), and 33%–50% of Asian and African EMs appear to have forms of the enzyme that are significantly less active than the form typically found in whites (Bertilsson et al. 1992; Sjoqvist et al. 1997; Smith and Mendoza 1996). Such individuals are sometimes referred to as SMs rather than PMs. In addition to genetic differences between various ethnic groups, some of the interethnic differences in enzyme activity may be due to a variety of environmental factors, such as diet, herbal medicines, and other lifestyle differences (Sjoqvist et al. 1997; Smith and Mendoza 1996).

CYP2C19 (mephenytoin hydroxylase) is also associated with marked interethnic differences. This enzyme metabolizes diazepam and several antidepressants (Pi and Gray 1998). Between 2% and 10% of whites have little or no activity of this enzyme, whereas 15%–25% of Asians may be PMs (Horai et al. 1989; Kupfer and Preisig 1984; Pi and Gray 1998). In addition, there is also evidence of polymorphism among EMs, with some Asian EMs having a form of the enzyme with less activity than that of the form commonly found in Caucasian EMs (Sjoqvist et al. 1997).

CYP3A4 (nifedipine oxidase) is involved in the metabolism of many psychotropic medications, including most benzodiazepines, several antidepressants (nefazodone, sertraline, and venlafaxine), and carbamazepine (Pi and Gray 1998). It appears that Asians have lower CYP3A4 activity than Caucasians have, but it is likely that these differences are due to diet or other environmental factors (Sjoqvist et al. 1997). This enzyme does not display polymorphism (Coutts 1994; Richelson 1997), but it is readily inducible (e.g., by carbamazepine and steroids), as well as inhibited by dietary compounds (e.g., by naringin, an ingredient of grapefruit juice). The interethnic differences in CYP3A4 activity likely are due to dietary differences or other environmental factors.

CYP1A2 (phenacetin O-deethylase) is responsible for the metabolism of clozapine and several other psychotropic medications, including some TCAs and tacrine (Pi and Gray 1998). Although there is considerable polymorphism, there are no consistent interethnic differences, with 12%–13% of whites, Asians, and Africans reportedly having little or no activity of this enzyme (Richelson 1997). The enzyme is highly inducible (e.g., by charbroiled beef, constituents of tobacco, industrial toxins, and cruciferous vegetables such as cabbage, broccoli, and cauliflower), so interethnic differences are certainly conceivable.

Finally, ethnic differences in plasma proteins that transport medications have also been found. Plasma concentrations of α1-acid glycoprotein, a plasma protein that provides binding sites for psychotropic drugs in the blood, are significantly lower in Asians than in Caucasians (Zhou et al. 1990).

Pharmacodynamics

Pharmacodynamics is concerned with the effect of a drug on the body, including tissue sensitivity or receptor binding. Pharmacokinetic differences between ethnic groups have received the most study, but pharmacodynamic differences have also been demonstrated.

One of the best-known examples involves the β-blocker propranolol. Asians not only require substantially lower doses of propranolol but also experience more effects of propranolol on blood pressure and heart rate. These differences are explained by pharmacodynamic factors (i.e., β-adrenoceptor sensitivity) not by pharmacokinetic factors (Zhou et al. 1989).

Some ethnic differences in therapeutic doses and side effects of various psychotropic medications, including neuroleptics, lithium, and TCAs, have also been explained by pharmacodynamic factors such as tissue or receptor sensitivity (Kalow 1989; Lin et al. 1995; Pi 1998).

Asian Culture and Attitudes Toward Mental Illness

More than half of the world's population is Asian, and the Asian population in the United States is increasing rapidly. The Asian American population nearly quadrupled between 1970 and 1990 (U.S. Bureau of the Census 1990). In 1990, the Asian population in the United States was 7.3 million, or more than 3% of the total United States population. It was projected that in the year 2000, the Asian population in the United States would be more than 12 million. Asian Americans are a very diverse ethnic, cultural, and linguistic group, comprising immigrants from many Asian countries as well as individuals born in the United States. For example, in the 1990 census (U.S. Bureau of the Census 1990), more than 20 Asian American ethnic groups were identified and it was found that 64% of Asian Americans were foreign born and 15% did not speak English well. Therefore, when assessing Asians in psychiatric practice, practitioners must make distinctions among specific Asian American groups and consider historical, social, and cultural differences.

Mental illness is frequently viewed as an embarrassment or stigma by Asian patients and their families. Asians tend to delay psychiatric care until they are seriously disturbed (Lin et al. 1982). When Asians do enter the mental health system, their psychiatric conditions often have become severe and chronic and likely require psychopharmacotherapy (Lin et al. 1982). Because Asians tend to underuse or avoid seeking psychiatric care, the general public and some health care professionals may believe that Asians are a well-adjusted "model minority" and have little or no need for psychiatric services. Consequently, there is a lack of culturally and linguistically competent treatment facilities and clinicians for Asian patients.

Culturally determined health beliefs and practices can also profoundly influence psychiatric assessment and psychopharmacotherapy. Cultural influences on symptoms manifested by Asian patients may mislead clinicians who are unfamiliar with Asian culture and health beliefs (Lin et al. 1995). For example, Asians are likely to express their problems in behavioral or somatic terms rather than in emotional ones. Also, Asian patients often present with somatic rather than psychological complaints and seek help from primary care physicians. However, findings from a recent epidemiological study of depressive disorders suggest that Chinese Americans are not adverse to expressing problems in emotional idioms (Takeuchi et al. 1998).

Even when modern, Western medical services are available, Asians frequently consider using indigenous or alternative remedies, and folk or traditional medicine may be tried first for treatment of a psychiatric disorder. Such treatment must be noted and monitored to avoid adverse drug interactions between traditional Asian herbal medicines and Western psychotropic medications. Also necessary is assessment of drug efficacy and toxicity, as well as placebo effects. Several studies have found that compliance with psychopharmacotherapy may be more problematic in non-Western than among Western populations. For example, Western medicines are believed to be more potent and more likely to cause side effects than are non-Western therapies, and interpretations and perceptions of side effects differ as well (Lee 1993; Smith et al. 1993).

Antipsychotics

There is a widespread impression that Asian patients require lower doses of antipsychotic medications than do white patients. Several retrospective surveys and studies have generally found that Asian patients received lower doses than Caucasians did, although the data are far from consistent (Pi and Gray 1998). For example, in a retrospective study involving 13 Asian and 13 white patients matched by age, sex, diagnosis, and chronicity, Lin and Finder (1983) found that Asians received about half the daily dose of antipsychotic that Caucasians received. However, both groups received relatively high average daily doses of antipsychotic (more than 1,000 mg chlorpromazine equivalents in Asians and more than 2,000 mg in whites). Ruiz et al. (1996) and Collazo et al. (1996) found lower doses being prescribed to Asians than to whites in the same public mental health system. Conversely, Sramek et al. (1986) failed to find such differences in the average daily doses of antipsychotics given to 30 Asian and 30 matched Caucasian patients.

During the 1980s, studies of prescribing practices in Asian countries indicated that physicians there prescribed dosages comparable to those used in the United States. In one such study, Pi et al. (1985) surveyed 29 medical schools in 9 countries regarding the prescribing practices and found dosages of antipsychotics to be essentially identical to those prescribed in the United States. However, it is difficult to know whether the dosages prescribed are truly reflective of the response of the individual patients to their medications. They may instead reflect prescribing patterns that either fail to acknowledge interindividual differences in dose (e.g., prescribing of the same standard dosage to all patients) or reflect presumed sensitivity of Asians to medications (resulting in prescribing of lower doses even in the absence of increased side effects).

Of more interest are well-controlled pharmacokinetic studies in which Asians have generally been found to have higher plasma concentrations of antipsychotics than those shown by Caucasians given the same weight-adjusted dose. For example, Potkin et al. (1984) gave haloperidol in doses of 0.4 mg/kg to 18 non-Asian American and 18 Chinese schizophrenic patients for 6 weeks and found the plasma haloperidol levels to be 52% higher in the Chinese patients than in the Americans. Similarly, Lin et al. (1988b), in a single-fixed-dose study, found that whites had lower serum haloperidol and prolactin concentrations than did American-born and foreign-born Asians. These authors suggested that the pharmacokinetic differences could at least partially explain the clinical impression that Asians may require lower doses of haloperidol than those required by whites to produce similar clinical effects. Such results are also consistent with the findings described earlier that a higher proportion of Asians have the CYP2D6 SM phenotype, because CYP2D6 is involved with the metabolism of haloperidol.

In a study of haloperidol and its metabolite, reduced haloperidol (reduction of the benzylic ketone C=O group to C-OH), it was found that reduced-haloperidol levels in Chinese patients were only about one-third those in age-matched non-Chinese patients (Jann et al. 1989). The lower reduced-haloperidol–to-haloperidol ratio in Chinese, caused either by a slower rate of reduction of haloperidol or a more active oxidation process converting reduced haloperidol back to haloperidol, could significantly affect the clearance of haloperidol and result in higher plasma levels of haloperidol.

A recent study of the atypical antipsychotic clozapine in Asians (Matsuda et al. 1996) found that Korean American patients showed a greater improvement than whites while receiving lower mean doses of clozapine. Korean Americans had lower mean clozapine concentrations than did Caucasians, yet they were more likely to experience anticholinergic and other side effects. No cases of agranulocytosis were reported in Korean American patients, and the incidence in Asians is not known. Clozapine is metabolized by CYP1A2, which is highly inducible, so such differences may be due to differences in diet and other personal habits.

Antipsychotic Medication–Induced Movement Disorders

Despite the important role of psychotropic medication–induced movement disorders (including extrapyramidal syndrome and tardive dyskinesia [TD]) in medication compliance, until recently ethnicity was little considered as a potential risk factor for these disorders, and most studies of the epidemiology of medication-induced movement disorders have ignored this variable (Gray and Pi 1998).

There is some evidence that Asians may be at increased risk of developing acute dystonic reactions. A retrospective review of records of 866 Chinese inpatients with schizophrenia revealed that

13% of the subjects had a history of developing acute dystonia when treatment with antipsychotic medications was first started, a figure somewhat higher than the rate of 2%–12% usually found in the United States (Ko et al. 1989). In a prospective study of ethnic differences in the development of acute extrapyramidal syndrome, 50% of Asian patients developed acute dystonia within the first 2 weeks of starting haloperidol therapy, whereas only 28% of white patients did so (Binder and Levy 1981). Although these two last percentages seem high, the doses of haloperidol (up to 70 mg/day) were also higher than those used today.

Less is known about the relationship between ethnicity and akathisia. In one study, 5% of Asian patients and 12% of white patients developed akathisia within the first 2 weeks of haloperidol therapy (Binder and Levy 1981). Because the number of patients studied was small, this difference was not statistically significant.

Whether Asians are at greater risk of antipsychotic-induced parkinsonism is also uncertain. In one study, Asian patients developed symptoms of parkinsonism while taking lower weight-adjusted doses and exhibiting lower serum haloperidol concentrations in comparison with Caucasian patients (Lin et al. 1989). In contrast, another study found little difference between Asians and whites, with 40% of Asian patients developing parkinsonism within 2 weeks of initiation of haloperidol therapy, compared with 35% of Caucasians (Binder and Levy 1981). In a study conducted in Japan (Binder et al. 1987), the prevalence of antipsychotic-induced parkinsonism was found to be 18%–40%, comparable to rates reported in the United States. Thus the data concerning Asians are contradictory.

The relationship between ethnicity and neuroleptic malignant syndrome (NMS) is unknown. In case reports and epidemiological studies, the age and sex of patients with NMS have typically been noted, but ethnicity has not. A study in China found that 0.63% of patients in whom treatment with antipsychotic medication was begun developed NMS (Deng et al. 1990), and an Indian study found 0.2% of patients developing the disorder (Singh 1981). These rates are similar to those found in American and European studies.

During the past four decades, there has been ongoing research into the epidemiology of TD. Only recently, however, have such studies included ethnicity as a variable (Gray and Pi 1998). The two most consistent risk factors associated with increased prevalence are advancing age and, to a lesser extent, female sex (Pi and Simpson 2000). If these are truly the consistent variables, there should not be significant differences between ethnic groups.

One approach to this issue would be to study the point prevalence of TD in various countries. Combining the results of published studies from Asian countries yields a prevalence of 11%, versus 28% from North American studies and 21% from European studies (Gray and Pi 1998). However, such an approach does not take into account differences in patient populations, methods of assessment, or definition of TD.

A better approach would be to compare studies conducted in different geographic regions by the same team of investigators, using the same diagnostic criteria. Using this approach, Ogita et al. (1975) studied 131 patients in France and 123 patients in Japan and found an equal prevalence of TD (18%) in the two populations.

In a larger investigation using this same design, Pi et al. (1993b) studied a total of 982 patients from 5 sites (Beijing, Yanji, and Hong Kong, China; Seoul, Korea; and Tottori, Japan). The prevalence of TD was 8% in Beijing, 19% among the Chinese in Yanji, 20% among the ethnic Koreans in Yanji, 19% in Hong Kong, 16% in Seoul, and 23% in Tottori. Even after controlling for age, sex, duration of illness, and antipsychotic dose, there was considerable variation between sites, with the sites other than Beijing having rates 1.9–2.9 times higher than in Beijing, a statistically significant difference. The similarity of TD prevalence among ethnic Chinese and Koreans in Yanji and the differences among ethnic Chinese between sites suggest that environmental factors (including prescribing practices), not genetic differences, were responsible for the variation.

Tan and Tay (1991) studied the prevalence of TD in Singapore among 514 patients age 60 years or more. In their study, the prevalence of TD among Asians was 28%, compared to 54% among Eurasians. Whether such variation was due to genetic or environmental factors was not clear.

The preferred method for studying the relationship between ethnicity and TD would be to study the incidence in a prospective cohort study involving a multiethnic population. No such study comparing Asians and Caucasians has been reported.

From the data reviewed here, it appears that Asian patients receiving antipsychotic medications are at increased risk of developing extrapyramidal syndrome. This would imply that Asians should receive lower doses of antipsychotics, because the antipsychotic effect of these medications occurs at a lower level of dopamine receptor blockade than does extrapyramidal syndrome. Reasons for the decreased risk of TD found in some studies are unclear but could include prescription of lower doses of antipsychotic medication or differences in either patient populations or methods of assessment.

Antidepressants

Much of the study of interethnic differences in the pharmacokinetics and pharmacodynamics of psychotropic medications has involved TCAs and differences between Asians and Caucasians (Pi et al. 1993a). As with antipsychotics, there are clinical reports that Asians require lower doses of TCAs (Pi and Gray 1998; Pi et al. 1993a). It has also been suggested that Asians show a therapeutic response at lower blood levels of TCAs (Yamashita and Asano 1979), suggesting pharmacodynamic differences. Other studies of prescribing patterns have failed to confirm this and found that the daily doses of amitriptyline, imipramine, doxepin, and nortriptyline prescribed by psychiatrists at 29 medical schools in 9 Asian countries were the same as those used in the United States (Pi et al. 1985). It was also reported that Asians and whites need similar doses of at least 150 mg/day to attain recommended therapeutic blood concentrations (Kinzie et al. 1987).

Desipramine is metabolized by CYP2D6. Given the high percentage of Asians who have the CYP2D6 SM phenotype (33%–50%), it would be expected that a greater percentage of Asians than Caucasians would metabolize desipramine slowly. Rudorfer et al. (1984) studied the pharmacokinetics of desipramine given as a single 100-mg oral dose in 14 Chinese and 16 white male and female physically and psychiatrically healthy volunteers. Asians had higher mean peak plasma desipramine levels than did Caucasians 8 hours after administration of the dose. Also, the peak plasma concentrations of the hydroxyl metabolite were higher in the Chinese population. No plasma protein–binding differences were found between the two groups. The Chinese subjects had significantly greater areas under the curve (AUCs) for both desipramine and its major metabolite, 2-hydroxydesipramine. The mean total plasma clearance of desipramine was higher in Caucasian than in Chinese subjects. Although most of the volunteers had intermediate rates of clearance, regardless of ethnicity, a few Chinese had slow clearance and a few whites had fast clearance, which led the investigators to propose a trimodal distribution of the desipramine clearance rate. The authors suggested that Asians who were SMs were at risk of toxicity from standard doses of TCAs. There was the suggestion that the differences were under genetic control.

Rudorfer et al. (1985) studied the kinetics of debrisoquin (a CYP2D6 substrate) given as a single 10-mg oral dose in 10 Chinese and 10 Caucasian volunteers, all but one of whom had participated in the desipramine study. The researchers were not able to demonstrate a relationship between the metabolism of the two drugs. Debrisoquin was cleared rapidly by every subject, including those who had shown slow clearance in the desipramine study. These results were difficult to explain, but one might speculate that desipramine is metabolized by a different enzyme or that some other step in the metabolic pathway results in the trimodal distribution of desipramine clearance. Given that relatively few Asians are CYP2D6 PMs but a high percentage of Asian EMs have a form of the enzyme that is less active than the form found in whites, the slower clearance of desipramine was most likely due to the SM form of the enzyme, rather than the PM form.

Pi et al. (1986) compared the pharmacokinetics of 50 mg desipramine in 20 Asian volunteers and 75 mg desipramine in 20 Caucasian volunteers of both sexes. Asians were found to achieve peak plasma concentrations in significantly less time (4.0 hours vs. 6.9 hours). No other pharmacokinetic parameters were found to be statistically significant between the two groups. Despite having the largest sample size for research of this kind, the authors noted that statistical confidence remained low.

Subsequently, Pi et al. (1989) undertook a more rigorously designed study (which included controlling for body weight [i.e., 1 mg desipramine per 1 kg body weight]) involving 18 Asian and 19 Caucasian age-matched healthy volunteers. The reverse of the previous result was found; the time required to achieve peak plasma concentrations was shorter in Caucasians (3.0 hours) than in Asians. The data also suggested the existence of a trimodal distribution of desipramine clearance in both Asians and Caucasians, with Asians having slightly fewer fast metabolizers. In the same study population, Pi et al. (1991) found no significant differences in the desipramine saliva-to-plasma ratio between Asian and Caucasian volunteers.

Kishimoto and Hollister (1984) conducted a pharmacokinetic study of single doses of 100 mg nortriptyline (in capsule form) in 10 American volunteers and 50 mg nortriptyline (in powdered suspension) in 10 Japanese volunteers. Japanese subjects achieved higher peak plasma concentrations and had a significantly higher mean AUC than did American subjects, a finding that the investigators interpreted as indicating a greater bioavailability of nortriptyline in the Japanese.

Koyama et al. (1996) evaluated the steady-state plasma levels of imipramine and desipramine in 28 Japanese patients with depression after they had received fixed doses of imipramine for a minimum of 2 weeks to phenotype for CYP2C19 metabolizer status. The authors found that the mean desipramine concentration–to-imipramine concentration ratio (*N*-demethylation index) was significantly reduced in patients who were designated PMs, compared with those who were designated EMs.

Clomipramine is also metabolized by CYP2D6 and CYP2C19. Given the high percentage of Asians who are CYP2D6 SMs (33%–50%) or CYP2C19 PMs (20%), it would be expected that a greater percentage of Asians than whites would metabolize clomipramine slowly. Allen et al. (1977) conducted a pharmacokinetic study of 25 mg or 50 mg clomipramine given as a single dose and found that 6 Asian Indian or Pakistani male volunteers had significantly higher mean plasma levels of clomipramine 4 hours after administration of the dose than did 11 English male volunteers. Also, Lewis et al. (1980) reported that at different time points up to 24 hours after treatment, the Pakistani/Indian group had higher peak plasma concentrations with the 50-mg dose and appeared to be more genuinely sensitive to adverse drug reactions.

Shimoda et al. (1995) studied 108 Japanese psychiatric patients, more than 80% of whom were experiencing a major depressive episode, and the results did not support the hypothesis that Asians metabolize clomipramine more slowly compared with people of other ethnicities or races. Clomipramine was titrated up to total doses ranging from 30 to 250 mg/day and was maintained at the same dose for 14 days before blood sampling was performed. At the conclusion of the analysis, apparent poor desmethylators, poor hydroxylators, or poor glucuronidators were not found. Negative findings such as this are to be expected, because there is considerable variability within ethnic groups in CYP activity, with not all members of a given ethnic group having the same CYP isozyme phenotypes.

As mentioned in two critical reviews on transcultural psychopharmacology of the TCAs (Pi et al. 1993a; Sramek and Pi 1999), the concept of differences between Asian and non-Asian populations in the pharmacokinetics and pharmacodynamics of TCAs has gained support from clinical reports and controlled studies. Whether these differences are due to ethnicity, pharmacokinetics, pharmacodynamics, environmental factors, or shortcomings of study design (such as small sample size) is not definitely known. Although recent studies of CYP polymorphism support the possibility of genetic differences, future studies will need to address these issues.

Monoamine oxidase inhibitors are not commonly prescribed to Asians, because many traditional Asian foods, including fermented bean curd, soy sauce, and fermented soybeans, contain relatively high levels of tyramine (a pressor amine), ranging from 0.02 to 43.0 μmol/g (Sung et al. 1986). Because the vast majority of Asians are fast acetylators (Whitford 1978), the metabolism of phenelzine may be increased in Asians, resulting in higher dose requirements than in Caucasians.

Selective serotonin reuptake inhibitors (SSRIs) are now widely prescribed for depression and other psychiatric disorders. The frequency of their use has already surpassed that for all other classes of antidepressants, but the possibility of ethnic variations in response has not yet been systematically studied.

There have been no pharmacokinetic studies of SSRIs and other newer antidepressants in which Asians and non-Asians were compared. Further research into the pharmacokinetics and pharmacodynamics of antidepressants, including these newer agents, among ethnic groups is necessary (Sramek and Pi 1996, 1999).

Benzodiazepines

In a survey involving 29 medical schools in 9 Asian countries, it was found that the doses of chlordiazepoxide, diazepam, lorazepam, and oxazepam used to treat acute anxiety were actually somewhat higher than those recommended in the United States, although maintenance doses were similar (Pi et al. 1985). As noted earlier, interpretation of such prescribing surveys requires caution.

In a study of benzodiazepine pharmacokinetics, it was found that the volume of distribution of diazepam was lower, and both serum diazepam and desmethyldiazepam levels were higher in Asian than in white physically and psychiatrically healthy volunteers (Ghoneim et al. 1981; Kumana et al. 1987). These pharmacokinetic differences became statistically insignificant after controlling for ethnic differences in skinfold thickness and the ratio of actual to ideal body weight, suggesting that ethnic differences might be due to differences in the percentage of body fat.

Lin et al. (1988a) examined plasma alprazolam concentrations and acute behavioral effects in 14 American-born Asian, 14 foreign-born Asian, and 14 Caucasian healthy male volunteers. Both Asian groups had greater AUCs and peak plasma concentrations and lower total plasma clearance than did the white group, after both oral and intravenous administration of alprazolam. There was no significant difference between the two Asian groups in any of the pharmacokinetic parameters examined. Pharmacodynamically, the only significant difference was that foreign-born Asians experienced more sedation compared with both Caucasian and American-born Asian subjects.

Ajir et al. (1997) reported that Asians had higher maximum serum concentrations, larger AUCs, and lower clearance of both adinazolam and its major active metabolite than did their Caucasian and African American counterparts. With oral administration, Asians also had higher maximum serum concentrations for both adinazolam and its metabolite. These findings support the concept that Asian patients require smaller doses of adinazolam than do white patients to achieve similar levels of adinazolam and its metabolite.

Lithium

Several surveys and case series suggest that Chinese and Japanese patients may respond to lower doses and plasma levels (0.3–0.9 mEq/L) of lithium than those commonly used to treat non-Asian populations (Pi and Gray 1998). For example, Chang et al. (1985) reported optimal therapeutic lithium concentrations of 0.71 and 0.73 mEq/L for Chinese patients with bipolar depression living in Shanghai and Taipei, respectively, compared with a mean level of 0.98 mEq/L for matched white American patients. This finding is in contrast to the belief held by medical school faculty in Asian countries that higher lithium levels are needed for effective treatment in the acute phase of mania (Pi et al. 1985). No significant differences in pharmacokinetics of lithium between ethnic groups have been found in controlled studies (Chang et al. 1985; Takahashi 1979; Yang 1985).

Recommendations and Conclusions

The increasing mobility of populations (including immigration) has resulted in our society's becoming more ethnically and culturally diverse than ever before. There has also been a growing interest in the impact of culture and ethnicity on the diagnosis and treatment of psychiatric disorders. Clinicians who treat ethnically and culturally diverse patient populations with mental disorders should be aware of the issues described so that they can tailor therapeutic regimens to best meet the needs of patients. An understanding of cross-cultural perspectives in psychopharmacology has become essential for psychiatrists who are treating increasing numbers of patients from different ethnic and socio-cultural backgrounds.

Systematic, scientifically designed studies of antipsychotics, lithium, antidepressants, and benzodiazepines have begun to probe the underlying mechanisms and clinical significance of pharmacogenetic, pharmacokinetic, and pharmacodynamic differences among various ethnic groups. Many questions regarding the cross-cultural aspects of psychotropic medications remain unanswered because of limitations in study design. Caution is required in interpreting findings, to avoid drawing conclusions based on a limited number of studies and on studies with methodological problems. To understand ethnicity and culture as significant influences on psychopharmacology, researchers must deal with definitions of ethnic populations, small sample size, factors affecting pharmacokinetic parameters, and pharmacodynamic considerations. It is necessary to apply standardized methods, enroll more representative subjects, and collect data on factors such as sex; age; lean and actual body weight; birthplace; residence; alcohol, nicotine, and caffeine intake; concomitant medical illness and medications; diet; menopausal status; menstrual cycle effects; and diagnosis and severity of psychiatric disorders. Also, careful monitoring is needed, to avoid the problems associated with large samples, particularly in multicenter studies. To the greatest extent possible, diagnostic criteria and rating and diagnostic techniques should be standardized and confirmed. Only then can it be known whether there truly are transcultural differences in response to psychotropic medications and, if such differences exist, can their causes be determined (Pi 1998; Pi and Gray 1998; Sramek and Pi 1999).

One simple explanation for the opinion generally held by psychiatrists that Asians require lower doses of medications may be bias on the part of the prescribers, who may think that Asians will respond to lower doses and hence only prescribe lower doses. This would explain why doses prescribed to Asians in the United States are often reported to be low and those prescribed in Asian countries are not (Pi 1998).

There may, however, be true differences in the metabolism of drugs between Asians and non-Asians, as recent studies of CYP phenotypes suggest. Whether such differences are due to genetics, environmental factors, or both needs to be assessed. Such differences in CYP isozymes affect metabolism of many psychotropic medications. Slower metabolism of psychotropic medications results in higher plasma drug levels, which can lead to a greater incidence of adverse side effects. Given the ethnic differences in CYP phenotypes, certain groups might require lower doses than others. The possibility of pharmacodynamic differences (e.g., differences in response to the same tissue concentration of the drug and different receptor sensitivity) also requires considerably more study. Furthermore, the impact of ethnicity and culture on dosing of newer antidepressant medications and atypical antipsychotics must be studied.

In conclusion, because metabolism of these drugs may vary by ethnic group (in addition to varying because of pharmacodynamic differences), understanding similarities and differences in cultures can play an important role in ensuring that patients receive optimum therapy and appropriate care. Until it is possible to predict which patients will be most sensitive to the effects of a given medication, the standard of practice should be applied for all ethnic groups—namely, prescription of the lowest dose needed to maximize therapeutic effects and minimize side effects.

References

Agarwal DP, Goedde HW: Alcohol metabolism, alcohol intolerance and alcoholism: biochemical and pharmacogenetic approaches. Berlin, Springer-Verlag, 1990

Ajir K, Smith M, Lin KM, et al: The pharmacokinetics and pharmacodynamics of adinazolam: multi-ethnic comparisons. Psychopharmacology 129:265–270, 1997

Allen JJ, Rack PH, Vaddadi KS: Differences in the effects of clomipramine on English and Asian volunteers: preliminary report on a pilot study. Postgrad Med J 53 (suppl 4):79–86, 1977

Bertilsson L, Lou YQ, Du YL, et al: Pronounced differences between native Chinese and Swedish populations in the polymorphic hydroxylations of debrisoquine and S-mephenytoin. Clin Pharmacol Ther 51:388–397, 1992

Binder RL, Levy R: Extrapyramidal reactions in Asians. Am J Psychiatry 138:1243–1244, 1981

Binder RL, Kazamatsuri H, Nishimura T, et al: Tardive dyskinesia and neuroleptic-induced parkinsonism in Japan. Am J Psychiatry 144: 1494–1496, 1987

Chang SS, Pandey GN, Yang YY, et al: Lithium pharmacokinetics: interracial comparison. Paper presented at the annual meeting of the American Psychiatric Association, Dallas, TX, May 19–24, 1985

Collazo Y, Tam R, Sramek J, et al: Neuroleptic dosing in Hispanic and Asian inpatients with schizophrenia. Mt Sinai J Med 63:310–313, 1996

Coutts RT: Polymorphism in the metabolism of drugs, including antidepressant drugs: comments on phenotyping. J Psychiatry Neurosci 19:30–44, 1994

Deng MZ, Chen GQ, Phillips MR: Neuroleptic malignant syndrome in 12 of 9,792 Chinese inpatients exposed to neuroleptics: a prospective study. Am J Psychiatry 147:1149–1155, 1990

Edeki T: Clinical importance of genetic polymorphism of drug oxidation. Mt Sinai J Med 63:291–300, 1996

Ghoneim MM, Korttila MK, Chian CK, et al: Diazepam effects and kinetics in Caucasians and Orientals. Clin Pharmacol Ther 29:749–756, 1981

Gonzalez FJ: Human cytochromes P450: problems and prospects. Trends Pharmacol Sci 13:346–352, 1992

Gray GE, Pi EH: Ethnicity and psychotropic medication related movement disorders. Journal of Practical Psychiatry and Behavioral Health 4:259–264, 1998

Horai Y, Nakano M, Ishizaki T, et al: Metoprolol and mephenytoin oxidation polymorphism in Far Eastern Oriental subjects: Japanese versus mainland Chinese. Clin Pharmacol Ther 46:198–207, 1989

Jann MW, Chang WH, Davis CM, et al: Haloperidol and reduced haloperidol plasma levels in Chinese vs. non-Chinese psychiatric patients. Psychiatry Res 30:45–52, 1989

Kalow W: Race and therapeutic drug response. N Engl J Med 320:588–589, 1989

Kalow W: Interethnic variation of drug metabolism. Trends Pharmacol Sci 12:102–107, 1991

Kinzie JD, Leung P, Boehnlein JK, et al: Antidepressant blood levels in Southeast Asians: clinical and cultural implications. J Nerv Ment Dis 175:480–485, 1987

Kishimoto A, Hollister LE: Nortriptyline kinetics in Japanese and Americans. J Clin Psychopharmacol 4:171–172, 1984

Ko GN, Zhang LD, Yan WW, et al: The Shanghai 800: prevalence of tardive dyskinesia in a Chinese psychiatric hospital. Am J Psychiatry 146:387–389, 1989

Koyama E, Tanaka T, Chiba K, et al: Steady-state plasma concentrations of imipramine and desipramine in relation to S-mephenytoin 4'-hydroxylation status in Japanese depressive patients. J Clin Psychopharmacol 16:286–293, 1996

Kroemer HK, Eichelbaum M: It's the genes, stupid: molecular basis and clinical consequences of genetic cytochrome P450 2D6 polymorphism. Life Sci 56:2285–2298, 1995

Kumana CR, Lauder IJ, Chan M, et al: Differences in diazepam pharmacokinetics in Chinese and white Caucasians: relation to body lipid stores. Eur J Clin Pharmacol 32:211–215, 1987

Kupfer A, Preisig R: Pharmacogenetics of mephenytoin: a new drug hydroxylation polymorphism in man. Eur J Clin Pharmacol 26:753–759, 1984

Lee S: Side effects of chronic lithium therapy in Hong Kong Chinese: an ethnopsychiatric perspective. Cult Med Psychiatry 17:301–320, 1993

Lewis P, Rack PH, Vaddadi KS, et al: Ethnic differences in drug response. Postgrad Med J 56(suppl 1):46–49, 1980

Lin K-M, Finder EJ: Neuroleptic dosage for Asians. Am J Psychiatry 140:490–491, 1983

Lin K-M, Innui TS, Kleinman A, et al: Sociocultural determinants of the help-seeking behavior of patients with mental illness. J Nerv Ment Dis 170:78–85, 1982

Lin K-M, Lau J, Smith M, et al: Comparison of alprazolam plasma levels and behavioral effects in normal Asian and Caucasian male volunteers. Psychopharmacology (Berl) 96:365–369, 1988a

Lin K-M, Poland RE, Lau JK, et al: Haloperidol and prolactin concentrations in Asians and Caucasians. J Clin Psychopharmacol 8:195–201, 1988b

Lin K-M, Poland RE, Nuccio I, et al: A longitudinal assessment of haloperidol doses and serum concentrations in Asian and Caucasian schizophrenic patients. Am J Psychiatry 146:1307–1311, 1989

Lin K-M, Anderson D, Poland RE: Ethnicity and psychopharmacology: bridging the gap. Psychiatr Clin North Am 18:635–647, 1995

Linder MW, Prough RA, Valdes R Jr: Pharmacogenetics: a laboratory tool for optimizing therapeutic efficiency. Clin Chem 43:254–256, 1997

Matsuda KT, Cho MC, Lin KM, et al: Clozapine dosage, serum levels, efficacy, and side-effect profiles: a comparison of Korean-American and Caucasian patients. Psychopharmacol Bull 32:253–257, 1996

Mucklow JC, Fraser HS, Bulpitt CJ, et al: Environmental factors affecting paracetamol metabolism in London factory and office workers. Br J Clin Pharmacol 10:67–74, 1980

Ogita K, Yazi G, Itoh H, et al: Comparative analysis of persistent dyskinesias of long-term usage with neuroleptics in France and in Japan. Folia Psychiatr Neurol Jpn 29:315–320, 1975

Pi EH: Transcultural psychopharmacology: present and future. Psychiatry Clin Neurosci 52:S185–S187, 1998

Pi EH, Gray GE: A cross-cultural perspective on psychopharmacology. Essential Psychopharmacology 2:233–262, 1998

Pi EH, Simpson GM: Medication-induced movement disorders, in Kaplan and Sadock's Comprehensive Textbook of Psychiatry, 7th Edition. Edited by Sadock BJ, Sadock VA. Philadelphia, PA, Lippincott Williams & Wilkins, 2000, pp 2265–2271

Pi EH, Jain A, Simpson GM: Review and survey of different prescribing practices in Asia, in Biological Psychiatry. Edited by Shagass C, Josiassen RC, Bridger WH, et al. New York, Elsevier, 1985, pp 1536–1538

Pi EH, Simpson GM, Cooper TB: Pharmacokinetics of desipramine in Caucasian and Asian volunteers. Am J Psychiatry 143:1174–1176, 1986

Pi EH, Tran-Johnson TK, Walker NR, et al: Pharmacokinetics of desipramine in Asian and Caucasian volunteers. Psychopharmacol Bull 25:483–487, 1989

Pi EH, Tran-Johnson T, Gray GE, et al: Saliva and plasma desipramine levels in Asian and Caucasian volunteers. Psychopharmacol Bull 27:281–284, 1991

Pi EH, Wang AL, Gray GE: Asian/Non-Asian transcultural tricyclic antidepressant psychopharmacology: a review. Prog Neuropsychopharmacol Biol Psychiatry 17:691–702, 1993a

Pi EH, Gutierrez MA, Gray GE: Tardive dyskinesia: cross-cultural perspectives, in Psychopharmacology and Psychobiology of Ethnicity. Edited by Lin K-M, Poland RE, Nakasaki G. Washington, DC, American Psychiatric Press, 1993b, pp 153–169

Potkin SG, Shen Y, Pardes H, et al: Haloperidol concentrations elevated in Chinese patients. Psychiatry Res 12:167–172, 1984

Richelson E: Pharmacokinetic drug interactions of new antidepressants: a review of the effects on the metabolism of other drugs. Mayo Clin Proc 72:835–847, 1997

Rudorfer MV, Lane EA, Chang WH, et al: Desipramine pharmacokinetics in Chinese and Caucasian volunteers. Br J Clin Pharmacol 17:433–440, 1984

Rudorfer MV, Lane EA, Potter WZ: Interethnic dissociation between debrisoquine and desipramine hydroxylation. J Clin Pharmacol 5:89–92, 1985

Ruiz S, Chu P, Sramek J, et al: Neuroleptic dosing in Asian and Hispanic outpatients with schizophrenia. Mt Sinai J Med 63:306–309, 1996

Shimoda K, Noguchi T, Ozeki Y, et al: Metabolism of clomipramine in a Japanese psychiatric population: hydroxylation, desmethylation, and glucuronidation. Neuropsychopharmacology 12:323–333, 1995

Singh G: The neuroleptic malignant syndrome. Indian Journal of Psychiatry 23:179–183, 1981

Sjoqvist F, Borga O, Dahl M-L, et al: Fundamentals of clinical pharmacology, in Avery's Drug Treatment, 4th Edition. Edited by Speight TM, Holford NHG. Auckland, Adis International, 1997, pp 1–73

Smith MW, Mendoza RP: Ethnicity and pharmacogenetics. Mt Sinai J Med 63:285–290, 1996

Smith MW, Lin K-M, Mendoza R: Nonbiological issues affecting psychopharmacotherapy: cultural considerations, in Psychopharmacology and Psychobiology of Ethnicity. Edited by Lin K-M, Poland RE, Nakasaki G. Washington, DC, American Psychiatric Press, 1993, pp 37–58

Sramek JJ, Pi EH: Ethnicity and antidepressant response. Mt Sinai J Med 63:320–325, 1996

Sramek JJ, Pi EH: Antidepressant response in ethnic populations, in Cross Cultural Psychiatry. Edited by Herrera JM, Lawson WB, Sramek JJ. New York, Wiley, 1999, pp 207–219

Sramek JJ, Sayles MA, Simpson GM: Neuroleptic dosage for Asians: failure to replicate. Am J Psychiatry 143:535–536, 1986

Sung SK, Lee CM, Young JD, et al: High levels of tyramine in some Chinese foodstuffs. Human Psychopharmacology 1:103–107, 1986

Takahashi R: Lithium treatment in affective disorders: therapeutic plasma level. Psychopharmacol Bull 15:32–35, 1979

Takeuchi DT, Chung RC-Y, Lin K-M, et al: Lifetime and twelve-month prevalence rates of major depressive episodes and dysthymia among Chinese Americans in Los Angeles. Am J Psychiatry 155:1407–1414, 1998

Tan CH, Tay LK: Tardive dyskinesia in elderly psychiatric patients in Singapore. Aust N Z J Psychiatry 25:119–122, 1991

U.S. Bureau of the Census: 1990 Summary Tape File 1C. Washington, DC, U.S. Bureau of the Census, 1990

Weber WW: The Acetylator Genes and Drug Responses. New York, Oxford University Press, 1987

Whitford GM: Acetylator phenotype in relation to monoamine oxidase inhibitor antidepressant drug therapy. International Pharmacopsychiatry 31:126–132, 1978

Yamashita I, Asano Y: Tricyclic antidepressants: therapeutic plasma level. Psychopharmacol Bull 15:40–41, 1979

Yang YY: Prophylactic efficacy of lithium and its effective plasma levels in Chinese bipolar patients. Acta Psychiatr Scand 71:171–175, 1985

Zhou HH, Koshakji RP, Silberstein DJ, et al: Altered sensitivity to and clearance of propranolol in men of Chinese descent as compared with American whites. N Engl J Med 320:565–570, 1989

Zhou HH, Adedoyin A, Wilkinson GR: Differences in plasma binding of drugs between Caucasians and Chinese subjects. Clin Pharmacol Ther 48:10–17, 1990

Chapter 5

Ethnopsychopharmacology in the Public Sector

Roy V. Varner, M.D.
Pedro Ruiz, M.D.
David R. Small, M.B.A.

The patient challenge faced by the general psychiatrist today is an increasing one, given the ever-evolving treatment strategies within the field of psychopharmacology. In this respect, the clinical challenge in recent years has become even greater for the practicing clinician as the field of ethnopsychopharmacology has evolved. During the past several decades, significant attention has been directed toward ethnopharmacology within general medicine, and attention to the field within psychiatry has also increased (Escobar and Tuason 1980; Kalow 1989; Lin and Finder 1983; Wood and Zhou 1991; Yamamoto and Lin 1995; Zhou et al. 1989).

Several factors have contributed to this situation. First, increased numbers of people have been immigrating to the United States, due in large measure to the liberalization of migration laws during the middle 1960s (Chien 1993; Ruiz 1993). Second, the last two or three decades have seen an increase in clinical recognition of cross-cultural psychiatry (Burnam et al. 1986; Gaw 1993; Gonzalez et al. 1995; Ruiz 1985). Additionally, contributions in the area of cross-cultural psychiatry have clearly demonstrated the role and the importance of race and ethnic factors in biopsychosocial research (Kleinman et al. 1978; Lin et al. 1993).

In this chapter, we attempt to ease some of the psychiatric practitioner's clinical challenges by presenting and discussing ethnopsychopharmacological data we derived from experience in the public sector. On the basis of findings from our recent retrospective ethnopsychopharmacological studies, which underline the importance of race or ethnic differences with respect to pharmacokinetics, pharmacodynamics, and pharmacogenetics, we hope to stimulate consideration of new conceptual models and research pathways relevant to psychiatric treatment of multiethnic populations in the public sector.

Ethnopsychopharmacological Background

Within general medicine, research into the response to nonpsychopharmacological treatments according to ethnicity or race has been conducted for some time (Benitez et al. 1988; Branch et al. 1978). In more recent years, psychopharmacological treatments and their relationship to ethnicity or race have begun to be studied (Lin 1992; Ruiz et al. 1999; Varner et al. 1998). The majority of this research focused initially on the response to neuroleptics (Lin and Finder 1983; Lin et al. 1988; Potkin et al. 1984) and lithium (Yang 1985) among Asian American patients. Additional research efforts have also focused on extrapyramidal reactions to neuroleptics among Asian American patients (Binder and Levy 1981; Yamamoto et al. 1979).

To a lesser degree, reports of studies of comparative dosing and response to psychopharmacological agents among Caucasian, African American, and Hispanic patients have begun to appear in the medical literature (Gaviria et al. 1986; Lin et al. 1986; Marcos and Cancro 1982; Mendoza et al. 1991; Strickland et al. 1991). Ziegler and Biggs (1977) reported that when African American and Caucasian patients were given comparable doses of amitriptyline and nortriptyline, the African Americans achieved higher levels and faster rates of clinical recovery. Moreover, it was also reported that African American patients had higher serum levels of tricyclic antidepressants (TCAs) than Caucasian patients did when measurements were made during periods after suicide attempts with drug overdoses (Rudorfer and Robbins 1982). In another study, African American male patients responded better to imipramine treatment than Caucasian patients did (Raskin et al. 1975). Still another research study suggested that TCAs produced delirium more commonly in African American patients than in Caucasian patients (Livingston et al. 1983).

Without question, research efforts in the field of ethnopsycho-pharmacology have been promising; however, more attention and further study are required. The data presented from our ethno-psychopharmacological studies are evidence of the current trend of focusing not only on traditional antidepressant agents (TCAs) and typical neuroleptics but also on selective serotonin reuptake inhibitor (SSRI) antidepressants and atypical neuroleptics or antipsychotics.

Houston Public Sector

The Harris County Psychiatric Center (HCPC) is the primary academic inpatient facility of the Department of Psychiatry and Behavioral Sciences of the University of Texas Medical School at Houston. Located on the campus of the Texas Medical Center, HCPC is Houston's largest psychiatric inpatient hospital and is almost fully devoted to a population identified primarily as indigent or receiving public financial assistance. In that sense, HCPC operates similarly to a state hospital. HCPC also has a close relationship with the ambulatory care programs of the Harris County Mental Health and Mental Retardation Authority. Additionally, HCPC plays an integral part in Houston's public sector continuum of psychiatric care.

HCPC has 250 beds and an average of about 5,000 admissions per year. The mean age of patients treated at HCPC is 36 years. The most common psychiatric disorders treated at HCPC are schizophrenia, other psychotic conditions, bipolar disorders, major depression, and other mood disorders. Many of these disorders are caused by substance abuse or are present in patients with substance abuse disorders or conditions.

When SSRIs were developed, we incorporated them into our ethnopsychopharmacological research. Initially, we compared patterns of use of the newer antidepressants with those of the older ones (TCAs). By the mid 1990s, it was becoming clear that SSRIs were rapidly replacing TCAs and other older antidepressant agents as drugs of first choice in the treatment of depression.

The multicultural character of both greater Houston and the patients at HCPC raised our interests in the possible ethnic differences in prescribing patterns of these newer drugs and in the dif-

Table 5–1. Probability of treatment with TCAs or SSRIs, by ethnicity

Ethnicity	TCAs (%)	SSRIs (%)	HCPC census (%)
Caucasian	44	56	45
African American	70	30	41
Hispanic	52	48	13
Asian American	33	67	1

Note. HCPC = Harris County Psychiatric Center; SSRI = selective serotonin reuptake inhibitor; TCA = tricyclic antidepressant.

ferences in responses to these newer drugs along ethnic lines. Using the pharmacy database of HCPC, we compared physicians' orders of TCAs with those of SSRIs by ethnic group (see Table 5–1).

The groups in Table 5–1 are the four major ethnic groups of patients treated at HCPC. Asian Americans make up the smallest of these groups. However, the data indicate that Asian American patients had the best chance of being prescribed SSRIs rather than TCAs. Additionally, African American patients were less likely than both Caucasian patients and Hispanic patients to be prescribed SSRIs. Moreover, Hispanics were less likely than Caucasian patients and more likely than African American patients to be prescribed SSRIs. It should be acknowledged that clinical factors other than prescribing patterns per se might have also contributed to these findings.

The next question was whether the pharmacy discharge profiles of our patients, sorted by ethnicity, would show differences in doses needed to produce clinical improvement sufficient to permit patient discharge.

Public Sector Studies

The data for our public sector studies were obtained from the HCPC pharmacy data system. Doses analyzed were study-drug doses administered on the day of discharge. The study years were 1994 for antidepressants, 1996 for typical neuroleptics, and 1997 and 1998 for atypical neuroleptics or antipsychotics. The patients selected for the antidepressant study included only those with a primary discharge diagnosis of nonpsychotic major depression

(DSM-III-R [American Psychiatric Association 1987], 296.2x and 296.3x). In the two neuroleptic or antipsychotic studies, the primary discharge diagnosis was restricted to schizophrenia (DSM-IV [American Psychiatric Association 1994], 295.xx). Diagnoses were made by HCPC medical staff on the basis of DSM-III-R and DSM-IV clinical criteria; drug selection and dosing were matters of attending physicians' clinical judgment. Discharge depended on attainment of the clinical improvement deemed appropriate for hospital discharge by the attending physician and documented in the treatment plan. Ethnicity was determined from the hospital's management information system database.

Patient exclusion criteria, which were common to all classes of drugs studied, were the following: age less than 18 years or more than 65 years, duplicate admissions during the study period, length of stay (LOS) of less than 7 days, adjunctive use of lithium or other augmenting psychopharmacological agents, and treatment with more than one drug within the study-drug classification. Also, when fewer than three patients were accrued within the same drug or ethnicity classification, those patients were excluded.

Dose, age, sex, LOS, and weight were tabulated for each patient in all drug studies.

Antidepressants

The selected sample of patients prescribed antidepressants consisted of 72 patients: 29 African Americans and 43 Caucasians (see Table 5–2). There were insufficient numbers of Hispanic and Asian American patients for inclusion of these ethnic groups in the study. Age and sex distributions are not shown in Table 5–2. The mean ages in the two patient groups were similar: 36.5 years for the African Americans and 35.1 years for the Caucasians. Male and female patients were nearly equally distributed in the two ethnic groups. The mean LOS for both Caucasian and African American patients treated with TCAs were about the same. However, among the patients given TCAs, the doses used to obtain the same levels of clinical response were higher in the Caucasian patient group.

Caucasian patients treated with desipramine or imipramine actually weighed slightly less than the corresponding African American patients. Therefore, one might have expected the Caucasian

Table 5–2. Antidepressants and ethnicity

	Caucasian	African American
TCAs		
No. of patients	21	11
LOS range (days)	7–34	7–34
Mean LOS (days)	19.1	18.7
Desipramine		
No. of patients	8	4
Dose range (mg)	150–400	50–250
Mean dose (mg)	234	150
Weight range (lb)	126–252	160–227
Mean weight (lb)	175	185
Imipramine		
No. of patients	4	4
Dose range (mg)	72–200	100–150
Mean dose (mg)	131	113
Weight range (lb)	116–150	84–194
Mean weight (lb)	133	142
Nortriptyline		
No. of patients	9	3
Dose range (mg)	50–125	75–100
Mean dose (mg)	92	83
Weight range (lb)	122–284	135–204
Mean weight (lb)	169	171
SSRIs		
No. of patients	22	18
LOS range (days)	7–32	8–33
Mean LOS (days)	20.7	19.0
Fluoxetine		
No. of patients	5	6
Dose range (mg)	20–40	20–40
Mean dose (mg)	24	26
Weight range (lb)	102–189	161–240
Mean weight (lb)	174	186

Table 5–2. Antidepressants and ethnicity *(continued)*

	Caucasian	African American
Sertraline		
No. of patients	17	12
Dose range (mg)	50–200	50–150
Mean dose (mg)	100	104
Weight range (lb)	92–265	119–241
Mean weight (lb)	154	184

Note. LOS = length of stay; SSRI = selective serotonin reuptake inhibitor; TCA = tricyclic antidepressant.

Source. Reprinted from Varner RV, Ruiz P, Small DR: "Black and White Patients' Response to Antidepressant Treatment for Major Depression." *Psychiatr Q* 69:117–125, 1998. Used with permission.

patients to require lower doses of TCAs than they received, to achieve levels of clinical response similar to those achieved by the African American patients. The weight difference between the two ethnic groups administered nortriptyline was negligible; however, Caucasian patients still received a higher mean dose of nortriptyline than did African American patients.

With regard to TCAs, Ziegler and Biggs (1977) reported that there were no differences in dosing between African American patients and Caucasian patients in one nortriptyline study. However, they also reported that African American patients had higher plasma levels of nortriptyline than did Caucasian patients, which suggests that African American patients might indeed require lower doses of TCAs when treated for major depression. This finding could help explain the lower doses of TCAs required in our African American patient sample. Along these lines, Livingston et al. (1983), in a study of TCA treatment of delirium, found higher levels of amitriptyline in African American patients than in Caucasian patients.

Amitriptyline was not among the TCAs in our study. However, the dosing patterns for all three TCAs in our patient samples suggest that African Americans may metabolize TCAs differently, perhaps because of genetic, physiologic, or environmental factors (Branch et al. 1978; Gonzales et al. 1995).

With regard to the SSRIs in our study (i.e., fluoxetine and sertraline), slightly lower mean doses were needed by Caucasian patients. However, there were notable differences in mean weight between these two patient groups; the Caucasians weighed considerably less than the African Americans. The mean weight difference should have predicted the need for a proportionally higher mean dose among African American patients. Therefore, when mean weight is taken into consideration, it appears that African Americans might need lower doses of SSRIs, compared with Caucasians, to achieve a similar clinical treatment outcome.

Neuroleptics or Antipsychotics

The selected sample of 204 patients receiving typical neuroleptics included 58 Caucasian, 135 African American, and 11 Hispanic patients. Eight neuroleptics were taken by these patients: chlorpromazine, thioridazine, thiothixine, loxapine, haloperidol, fluphenazine, perphenazine, and trifluoperazine. A haloperidol-equivalent dose was chosen as the basis of comparison for all eight typical neuroleptics included in this study. All 11 Hispanics received haloperidol. The results of this study are shown in Table 5–3.

Table 5–3. Typical neuroleptics and ethnicity

	Caucasian	African American	Hispanic
No. of patients	58	135	11
No. of male patients	44	82	7
No. of female patients	14	53	4
Age range (years)	18–65	21–62	23–56
Mean age (years)	41.4	37.5	35.2
LOS range (days)	8–42	7–60	9–26
Mean LOS (days)	19.7	18.6	14.5
Weight range (lb)	99–234	99–293	106–225
Mean weight (lb)	160	172	150
Dose range (mg)[a]	4–60	1–60	2–15
Mean dose (mg)[a]	16.2	15.5	7.6

Note. LOS = length of stay.
[a]Haloperidol equivalent.
Source. Reprinted from Ruiz P, Varner RV, Small DR, et al.: "Ethnic Differences in the Neuroleptic Treatment of Schizophrenia." *Psychiatr Q* 70:163–170, 1999. Used with permission.

The mean LOS for Caucasian patients and African American patients were similar (19.7 and 18.6 days, respectively), but the mean LOS for Hispanic patients was somewhat lower (14.5). African Americans had the highest mean weight (172 lb), 12 lb higher than that of the Caucasian patient group and 22 lb higher than that of the Hispanic patient group. The mean doses of typical neuroleptics in the Caucasian and African American patient groups were similar (16.2 mg and 15.5 mg, respectively), but the mean dose was considerably lower in the Hispanic patient group (7.6 mg). One could raise the question of haloperidol's having a unique effect in the Hispanic patient group, given that all 11 Hispanics received this drug. However, the majority of both Caucasian (58.6%) and African American patients (59.8%) also received haloperidol, minimizing this possibility.

Given the relatively small differences in mean weight between Caucasian patients and African American patients, mean doses of typical neuroleptics needed to obtain similar levels of clinical response in the treatment of schizophrenia in Caucasian and African American patients appear to have been quite similar. This finding contrasts with findings of previous studies that showed a prescribing bias toward higher doses of antipsychotic or neuroleptic drugs for African American patients compared with Caucasian patients (Segal et al. 1996; Yamamoto and Lin 1995). However, the amount of typical neuroleptics needed by Hispanics was dramatically less in those studies and in our study.

The results of a similar study of ours, in which the study drugs were three atypical neuroleptics or antipsychotics, are given in Table 5–4. During the time of this study, clozapine, olanzapine, and risperidone were the only atypical neuroleptic or antipsychotic agents in general use at HCPC; these three drugs were selectively used in accordance with the clinical criteria set by the Harris County Mental Health and Mental Retardation Authority. These criteria included documentation of at least two failures to respond clinically to treatment with different typical neuroleptic agents.

With respect to the atypical neuroleptic clozapine, the mean dose among African American patients (428.6 mg) compared with that for Caucasian patients (365.0 mg) suggests that African Americans need a higher mean dose of clozapine than do Cau-

Table 5–4. Atypical neuroleptics or antipsychotics and ethnicity

	Caucasian patients	African American patients	Hispanic patients	Asian American patients
Clozapine				
No. of patients	5	7	0	0
No. of male patients	2	5	0	0
No. of female patients	3	2	0	0
LOS range (days)	7–53	10–62	—	—
Mean LOS (days)	23.0	30.0	—	—
Age range (years)	23–48	26–55	—	—
Mean age (years)	38.6	38.0	—	—
Dose range (mg)	75–500	300–600	—	—
Mean dose (mg)	365.0	428.6	—	—
Weight range (lb)	126–292	148–252	—	—
Mean weight (lb)	181.6	182.6	—	—
Olanzapine				
No. of patients	14	18	3	3
No. of male patients	8	10	1	1
No. of female patients	6	8	2	2
LOS range (days)	7–33	7–48	7–21	8–32
Mean LOS (days)	17.7	16.5	13.3	16.3
Age range (years)	22–62	25–65	33–58	28–42
Mean age (years)	40.4	43.6	45.0	36.3
Dose range (mg)	5–20	10–20	10–20	10
Mean dose (mg)	12.5	14.4	13.3	10.0
Weight range (lb)	137–244	114–250	161–196	138–180
Mean weight (lb)	174.2	187.6	179.0	159.7
Risperidone				
No. of patients	21	32	6	0
No. of male patients	15	22	3	0
No. of female patients	6	10	3	0
LOS range (days)	7–41	7–47	8–36	—
Mean LOS (days)	16.0	18.6	15.2	—
Age range (years)	21–55	19–64	20–60	—
Mean age (years)	35.8	36.6	33.8	—
Dose range (mg)	1–12	2–8	2–8	—
Mean dose (mg)	5.6	4.8	4.0	—
Weight range (lb)	132–322	121–263	100–278	—
Mean weight (lb)	204.9	168.5	189.3	—

Note. LOS = length of stay.

casians. This impression is reinforced by the fact that the two groups had nearly identical mean weights (182.6 and 181.6 lb, respectively) and that African American patients stayed in the hospital 1 week longer.

In terms of the atypical antipsychotic olanzapine, a higher mean dose for African American patients (14.4 mg) than for Caucasian patients (12.5 mg) was again found. However, among patients receiving olanzapine, African Americans' mean weight was 13.4 lb higher than that of Caucasians. This mean weight difference might partially explain the impression that African American patients need a higher mean dose of olanzapine than Caucasian patients do. The mean dose required by Hispanic patients was intermediate between those required by African American and Caucasian patients. Additionally, the Hispanics' mean weight was 8.6 lb less and the mean LOS 3.2 days shorter than those of African American patients. The present data suggest that both Hispanics and African Americans might require higher mean doses of olanzapine compared with Caucasians. The mean dose required by the Asian American patients was dramatically lower (10.0 mg) than that required by any of the other three ethnic groups. Additionally, the mean weight of Asian Americans was much lower. Therefore, the data suggest that Asian Americans might need the lowest mean dose of olanzapine, because their dose-to-weight ratio is the lowest compared with the ratios in the other three ethnic groups studied.

Among patients receiving risperidone, Hispanics required only 4.0 mg to achieve a clinical response that permitted hospital discharge, compared with 4.8 mg for African Americans and 5.6 mg for Caucasians. These results are somewhat confounded by remarkable differences in mean weight between the three patient groups, with the Caucasian patients being the heaviest (204.9 lb), African American patients the lightest (168.5 lb), and Hispanic patients in between (189.3 lb). The Hispanic patients had the lowest dose-to-weight ratio, which suggests that Hispanics may need a lower risperidone mean dose than that required by Caucasian or African American patients. Caucasian and African American dose-to-weight ratios were similar, and thus the finding of a lower required mean dose for African Americans is less conclusive.

Discussion

Although research efforts in the field of ethnopharmacology have been limited, it is increasingly clear that medication dosing may be significantly affected by ethnic differences related to the pharmacodynamics, pharmacokinetics, and pharmacogenetics of certain medications. Fortunately, the literature on this subject is steadily proliferating.

The results of our study focusing on antidepressant dosing at the time of discharge tend to corroborate previous evidence that African American patients need lower doses of TCAs than do Caucasian patients. Results are more equivocal with respect to our study of African American and Caucasian patients taking SSRIs. However, when weight is taken into consideration, it is found that African Americans might need lower doses of SSRIs compared with Caucasians.

Among study patients receiving typical neuroleptic agents, there appeared to be little, if any, difference between African American and Caucasians. However, the data suggest that Hispanics need a considerably lower dose of typical neuroleptic agents than do either African Americans or Caucasians.

Findings of our study of atypical neuroleptics and antipsychotics show that African American patients may need a higher dose of clozapine than that required by Caucasian patients. Likewise, it appears that African Americans may need a higher dose of olanzapine than Caucasians do and that Hispanics have intermediate requirements. Asian patients appear to require the lowest dose of all, but it must be noted that the study included a relatively small sample of Asians. Finally, Hispanics may need a lower dose of risperidone than that required by African Americans or Caucasians, and the dose difference between the latter two groups may be negligible.

Conclusion

During the last 10–15 years, the field of neuroscience has gained much momentum and a considerable amount of new knowledge has been amassed. This growth in the neurosciences has also produced much stimulus and attention in the field of ethnopsychopharmacology. Besides, United States society is rapidly becoming pluralistic and multiethnic. Also, it is primarily in the public sector that these multicultural and multiethnic populations tend to receive their psychiatric care. Therefore, we decided to give priority to ethnopsychopharmacological research efforts in our public psychiatric hospital, the Harris County Psychiatric Center. We hope that the studies described in this chapter will further stimulate attention to the field of ethnopsychopharmacology, particularly in the public sector, ethnic minority groups, and gender-related populations.

References

American Psychiatric Association: Diagnostic and Statistical Manual of Mental Disorders, 3rd Edition, Revised. Washington, DC, American Psychiatric Association, 1987

American Psychiatric Association: Diagnostic and Statistical Manual of Mental Disorders, 4th Edition. Washington, DC, American Psychiatric Association, 1994

Benitez J, Llerena A, Cobaleda J: Debrisoquin oxidation polymorphism in a Spanish population. Clin Pharmacol Ther 44:74–77, 1988

Binder RL, Levy R: Extrapyramidal reactions in Asians. Am J Psychiatry 138:1243–1244, 1981

Branch RA, Salih SY, Homeida M: Racial differences in drug metabolizing ability: a study with antipyrine in the Sudan. Clin Pharmacol Ther 24:283–286, 1978

Burnam MA, Hough RL, Karno M: Acculturation and lifetime prevalence of psychiatric disorders among Mexican Americans in Los Angeles. J Health Soc Behav 28:89–102, 1986

Chien C: Ethnopsychopharmacology, in Culture, Ethnicity and Mental Illness. Edited by Gaw AC. Washington, DC, American Psychiatric Press, 1993, pp 413–430

Escobar JI, Tuason VB: Antidepressant agents: a cross-cultural study. Psychopharmacol Bull 16:49–52, 1980

Gaviria M, Gil AA, Javaid JI: Nortriptyline kinetics in Hispanic and Anglo subjects. J Clin Psychopharmacol 6:227–231, 1986

Gaw A (ed): Cross-Cultural Psychiatry. Washington, DC, American Psychiatric Press, 1993

Gonzalez CA, Griffith EEH, Ruiz P: Cross-cultural issues in psychiatric treatment, in Treatment of Psychiatric Disorders, 2nd Edition. Edited by Gabbard GO. Washington, DC, American Psychiatric Press, 1995, pp 55–74

Kalow W: Race and therapeutic drug response. N Engl J Med 320:588–589, 1989

Kleinman A, Eisenberg L, Good B: Clinical issues from anthropologic and cross-cultural research. Ann Intern Med 88:251–258, 1978

Lin K-M: Ethical aspects of psychopharmacological studies in different ethnic groups. Clinical Psychopharmacology 15:483A–484A, 1992

Lin K-M, Finder E: Neuroleptic dosage for Asians. Am J Psychiatry 140:490–491, 1983

Lin K-M, Poland RE, Lesser IM: Ethnicity and psycho-pharmacology. Cult Med Psychiatry 10:151–165, 1986

Lin K-M, Poland RE, Lau J, et al: Haloperidol and prolactin concentrations in Asians and Caucasians. J Clin Psychopharmacol 8:195–201, 1988

Lin K-M, Poland RE, Nakasaki G (eds): Psychopharmacology and Psychobiology of Ethnicity. Washington, DC, American Psychiatric Press, 1993

Livingston RL, Zucker D, Isenberg K, et al: Tricyclic antidepressants and delirium. J Clin Psychiatry 44:173–176, 1983

Marcos LR, Cancro R: Pharmacotherapy of Hispanic depressed patients: clinical observations. Am J Psychother 36:505–513, 1982

Mendoza R, Smith MW, Poland RE, et al: Ethnic psychopharmacology: the Hispanic and the Native American perspective. Psychopharmacol Bull 27:449–461, 1991

Potkin SG, Shen Y, Pardes H, et al: Haloperidol concentrations elevated in Chinese patients. Psychiatric Research 12:167–172, 1984

Raskin A, Thomas H, Crook MA: Antidepressants in black and white inpatients: differential response to a controlled trial of chlorpromazine and imipramine. Arch Gen Psychiatry 32:643–649, 1975

Rudorfer MJ, Robbins ELI: Amitriptyline overdose: clinical effects on tricyclic antidepressant plasma levels. J Clin Psychiatry 43:457–460, 1982

Ruiz P: Cultural barriers to effective medical care among Hispanic-American patients. Annu Rev Med 36:63–71, 1985

Ruiz P: Access to health care for uninsured Hispanics: policy recommendations. Hospital and Community Psychiatry 44:958–962, 1993

Ruiz P, Varner RV, Small DR, et al: Ethnic differences in the neuroleptic treatment of schizophrenia. Psychiatr Q 70:163–170, 1999

Segal SP, Bola JR, Watson MA: Race, quality of care, and antipsychotic prescribing practices in psychiatric emergency services. Psychiatr Serv 47:282–286, 1996

Strickland TL, Ranganath V, Lin KM, et al: Psychopharmacologic considerations in the treatment of black American populations. Psychopharmacol Bull 27:441–448, 1991

Varner RV, Ruiz P, Small DR: Black and white patients' response to antidepressant treatment for major depression. Psychiatr Q 69:117–125, 1998

Wood AJJ, Zhou HH: Ethnic differences in drug disposition and responsiveness. Clin Pharmacokinet 20:1–24, 1991

Yamamoto J, Lin KM: Psychopharmacology, ethnicity and culture, in American Psychiatric Press Review of Psychiatry, Vol 14. Edited by Oldham JM, Riba MB. Washington, DC, American Psychiatric Press, 1995, pp 529–541

Yamamoto J, Fung D, Lo S, et al: Psychopharmacology for Asian Americans and Pacific Islanders. Psychopharmacol Bull 15:29–31, 1979

Yang YY: Prophylactic efficacy of lithium and its effective plasma levels in Chinese bipolar patients. Acta Psychiatr Scand 71:171–175, 1985

Zhou HH, Koshakji RP, Silberstein DJ, et al: Altered sensitivity to and clearance of propranolol in men of Chinese descent as compared with American whites. N Engl J Med 320:565–570, 1989

Ziegler VE, Biggs JT: Tricyclic plasma levels: effects of age, race, sex and smoking. JAMA 238:2167–2169, 1977

Afterword

Pedro Ruiz, M.D.

The five chapters of this book represent the state of the art as far as ethnicity and psychopharmacology are concerned. The field of ethnopsychopharmacology has benefited from the emphasis given in recent years to the neurosciences. Research efforts in the neurosciences, which have produced a considerable amount of new knowledge in the last two decades, have stimulated and given recognition to the field of ethnopsychopharmacology.

The recent advances in ethnopsychopharmacology are, we believe, beneficial to the United States. The country is becoming more and more pluralistic and multiethnic (Alarcon and Ruiz 1995; Gonzalez et al. 1995). As different ethnic or cultural groups grow in the United States, attention needs to be given to the way in which these populations manifest psychiatric symptoms and to the groups' conceptions of the etiology of mental illness and their ability to obtain psychiatric care, as well as to the unique pharmacokinetics, pharmacodynamics, and pharmacogenetics among these populations (Ruiz 1993, 1998a, 1998b; Ruiz et al. 1995; Ware et al. 1996). If this attention is lacking, frustration in both patients and psychiatric practitioners will develop, misdiagnoses will be made, treatment errors will occur, and, more important, noncompliance with treatment will become highly prevalent (Kleinman et al. 1978; Ruiz 1985, 1995; Ruiz and Ruiz 1983).

In many ways, the current attention given to ethnopsychopharmacology has not only clinical relevance but also educational relevance. At present, there is a focus on evidence-based medicine and the development of core competencies. Research efforts in the field of ethnopsychopharmacology will be useful in this respect.

We think this book is very timely. In the twenty-first century, we expect to see further globalization of psychiatry as well as of society. As this happens, cross-cultural psychiatry will become even more relevant, as will ethnopsychopharmacology. The scientific advances achieved in recent years in ethnopsychopharmacology have set the stage for much scientific growth in this field in the near future. It is to be hoped that this book will be a strong stimulus in this regard.

We hope that the readers of this book have found the contributions well integrated, balanced, original, and challenging. It was our aim to create interest in this subject and to stimulate further reading. We hope this book will be helpful to psychiatric practitioners in their day-to-day clinical practices and useful to educators and investigators in their academic pursuits.

References

Alarcon RD, Ruiz P: Theory and practice of cultural psychiatry in the United States and abroad, in American Psychiatric Press Review of Psychiatry, Vol 14. Edited by Oldham JM, Riba MB. Washington, DC, American Psychiatric Press, 1995, pp 599–626

Gonzalez CA, Griffith EEH, Ruiz P: Cross-cultural issues in psychiatric treatment, in Treatments of Psychiatric Disorders, 2nd Edition, Vol 1. Edited by Gabbard GO. Washington, DC, American Psychiatric Press, 1995, pp 55–85

Kleinman A, Eisenberg L, Good B: Culture, illness, and care: clinical lessons from anthropologic and cross-cultural research. Ann Intern Med 88:251–258, 1978

Ruiz P: Cultural barriers to effective medical care among Hispanic-American patients. Annu Rev Med 36:63–71, 1985

Ruiz P: Access to health care for uninsured Hispanics: policy recommendations. Hospital and Community Psychiatry 44:958–962, 1993

Ruiz P: Assessing, diagnosing, and treating culturally diverse individuals: a Hispanic perspective. Psychiatr Q 66:329–341, 1995

Ruiz P: New clinical perspectives in cultural psychiatry. Journal of Practical Psychiatry and Behavioral Health 4:150–156, 1998a

Ruiz P: The role of culture in psychiatric care. Am J Psychiatry 155:1763–1765, 1998b

Ruiz P, Ruiz PP: Treatment compliance among Hispanics. Journal of Operational Psychiatry 14:112–114, 1983

Ruiz P, Venegas-Samuels K, Alarcon RD: The economics of pain: mental health care costs among minorities. Psychiatr Clin North Am 18:659–670, 1995

Ware JE, Bayliss MS, Rogers WH, et al: Differences in 4-year health outcomes for elderly and poor, chronically ill patients treated in HMO and fee-for-service systems. JAMA 276:1039–1047, 1996

Index

*Page numbers printed in **boldface** type refer to tables or figures.*

Anxiety disorders in African Americans, 39–41
Asian Indians
    compliance with treatment among, 7
    drug metabolism in, 21
Asians, xix, 91–113
    on antidepressants, 101–105
    on antipsychotics, 96–101
        dosage, 96–97
        movement disorders induced by, 98–101
    on benzodiazepines, 105–106
    culture and attitudes toward mental illness, 95–96
    CYP2C19 metabolism in, 19
    CYP2D6 genotyping of, 61
    dextromethorphan metabolic ratios (MRs) in, **18**
    dosing of, 42
    extensive metabolism in, 61
    on lithium, 106
    perception of drug effects, 8
    pharmacogenetic findings in, 61–63
    public sector study of, 124
    response to levodopa, 24
    on SSRIs vs. TCAs, **118**
Azarcon, 68

Benzodiazepines, Asians on, 105–106
Bias, physician, xvii
Biodiversity, psychotropic responses and, 12–24
Bipolar affective disorder, 38
Black patients, compliance with treatment among, 7. *See also* African Americans

Carbamazepine, 44

Catecholamines, 23
Catechol *O*-methyltransferase (COMT), 23–24
Caucasians
    CYP2C19 metabolism in, 19
    dextromethorphan metabolic ratios (MRs) in, **18**
    public sector study of, 117–125
        on neuroleptics or antipsychotics, **122,** 122–125, **124**
        on SSRIs vs. TCAs, **118**
Clinician attitudes, culture and, 5–6
Clinician-patient relationship, 4
Clomipramine, 103–104
Clozapine, 45, 73, 79, 123–125, **124**
    Asians on, 98
Cold-hot balance in traditional medicine, 10
Color-blind approach, pitfall of, 2–3
Comfrey, 68
Commitment, African Americans' fear of involuntary, 39
Competitive inhibition, 67
Complementary medicine, xiii
Compliance. *See* Adherence (compliance)
Concomitant medications, 10–12, 66–67, 81
Cultural context, 1–36
    adherence (compliance) and, 4, 6–8
    alternative/indigenous/ traditional medicine and, 9–12

Quercetin, 66

Races, xv
Receptors, genetic
polymorphism of genes
encoding, 21–23, 26
Red blood cell–to-plasma ratio,
43–44
Refugee patients, compliance
among, 7
Responses to drugs. *See also*
Drug-metabolizing enzymes
biodiversity and, 12–14
factors affecting, **3**
integrating culture and
biology to improve, 74–79
Rifampin, 67
Risperidone, 45–46, 73–74, 123,
124, 125

Saudi Arabians, superextensive
metabolism in, 62
Schizophrenia, 22
in African Americans, 41–42
misdiagnosis of, 37, 38, 39
in Hispanics, misdiagnosis of,
75–76
racial bias in diagnosis of, 5
Selective serotonin reuptake
inhibitors (SSRIs), 43, 105
Hispanics on, 71–72
public sector study of, **120,**
121–122
Serotonin, 21
Serotonin transporter gene
(5-HTT), 22–23
Sertraline, public sector study of,
121
Sex influences on
pharmacokinetics and
pharmacodynamics, 25–26

Siete azahares, 68–69
Signal transduction cascade,
24
Slow metabolizers (SMs), 93
Smoking, serum concentration of
psychotropics and, 20
Spaniards, pharmacogenetic
findings in, 61–63
SSRIs (selective serotonin
reuptake inhibitors), 43, 105
Steroid hormones, 26
Superextensive metabolism,
17–18, 62
Susto, 68

Tardive dyskinesia (TD), 44–45,
100–101
racial bias in diagnosis of, 5
TCAs. *See* Tricyclic
antidepressants
Terfenadine, 20
Traditional medical theories and
practices, 9–12
Transporters, genetic
polymorphism of genes
encoding, 21–23, 26
Trazodone, 70
Tricyclic antidepressants (TCAs),
117–118
African Americans on,
42–43
Asians on, 101–104
compliance with prescription
of, 7
Hispanics on, 69–71
public sector study of, **120,**
121
Tryptophan hydroxylase, 23
Tuberculosis, in Hispanics, 67
Tuskegee study, 46
Tyrosine hydroxylase, 23